D1413197

Things No Longer There

Things No Longer There

List $19.95
Discount $15.96

Purchased by_____

Things No Longer There

A Memoir of Losing Sight and Finding Vision

Susan Krieger

THE UNIVERSITY OF WISCONSIN PRESS

TERRACE BOOKS

The University of Wisconsin Press
1930 Monroe Street
Madison, Wisconsin 53711

www.wisc.edu/wisconsinpress/

3 Henrietta Street
London WC2E 8LU, England

1   3   5   4   2

Printed in the United States of America

Library of Congress Cataloging-in-Publication Data
Krieger, Susan.
Things no longer there: a memoir of losing sight and
finding vision / Susan Krieger.
p.   cm.
Includes bibliographical references.
ISBN 0-299-20864-8 (pbk.: alk. paper)
1. Krieger, Susan.   2. Lesbians—California—Biography.
3. Feminists—Biography.   4. Lesbian couples—Family relationships.
5. Aging.   6. Vision disorders.   I. Title.
HQ75.4.K75A3   2005
306.76′63′092—dc22   2004024546

Terrace Books, a division of the University of Wisconsin Press, takes its name
from the Memorial Union Terrace, located at the University of Wisconsin–Madison.
Since its inception in 1907, the Wisconsin Union has provided a venue for students,
faculty, staff, and alumni to debate art, music, politics, and the issues of the day.
It is a place where theater, music, drama, dance, outdoor activities, and
major speakers are made available to the campus and the community.
To learn more about the Union, visit www.union.wisc.edu.

For Estelle

Contents

Contents

Preface

Things No Longer There draws from my personal experiences to elaborate on a theme of losing sight and finding vision. I wrote this book during 1994–2003 and 1979–80, two periods of emotional significance in my life. Over the years, a core set of friends and colleagues have read these stories and given me responses which have improved each one and encouraged the whole. For devoted readings of the entire manuscript and for nurturing my spirit, I would like to thank Zandra Contaxis, Estelle Freedman, Paola Gianturco, and Carolyn Hallowell. For valuable responses to individual chapters and for encouraging me, I thank: Rhoda Cahn, Laura Carstensen, Pat Holt, Martin Krieger, Pat Mills, Leila Rupp, Terry Ryan, and Verta Taylor. At a crucial time, Peggy Pascoe read the manuscript and provided insightful comments on the novella section.

Several thoughtful editors guided me along the way. I am especially grateful to Norman Denzin for his generosity in reviewing this work and championing its publication. Two anonymous readers for the University of Wisconsin Press gave invaluable feedback and suggestions. I am indebted to my editor Raphael Kadushin for accepting the book and believing in its value. Susanne Breckenridge provided sensitive copyediting that enhanced the text. Sheila Moermond offered wise counsel during the publication process.

Each of the stories in *Things No Longer There* is an embroidery upon life; it is my take at a particular time, my account of an experience also shared with others. I am certain that those others who appear in these pages would tell quite different stories of the same experience. For sharing their lives with me and encouraging my writing, even though in the end, I would tell it my own way, I thank: Marythelma Brainard, Jane Jarrett, Kathe Morse, Richard Morse, Donna Humble, Kathy Vanozzi, Phoebe Wood, and the students in my classes at Stanford University.

In offering this book, I would like to honor the memory of Carolyn Hallowell, my psychotherapist for eighteen years, who died before she could see *Things No Longer There* come to fruition. Carolyn was with me from the very first paragraph I wrote. After reading it, she smiled at me and said, "It's going to be good." Wherever you are, Carolyn, thank you.

Most of all, I would like to thank Estelle Freedman, who shared so many of the experiences I describe and who, when my eyesight faded, threatening my sense of my ability to write, sprang into action and read my writing aloud to me so that I might begin to rekindle my confidence. This book may be about lost sight and things no longer there, but Estelle has been very present for me, never lost, never fading into a hazy landscape, but looking with me at these changing scenes and delighting with me in my sense of triumph in resurrecting them. Estelle, may we continue to lead one another with our different kinds of sight.

Things No Longer There

Introduction

THIS BOOK IS ABOUT THINGS no longer there in the outer world that are still very present in the mind. In it, I explore the way outer landscapes may change but inner visions of them persist, giving meaning, jarring the senses with a very different picture from what appears before the eyes. *Things No Longer There: A Memoir of Losing Sight and Finding Vision* is a culmination of my desire to paint with inner pictures the scenes, memories, and emotions, the invisible landscapes that illuminate my mind long after they have disappeared in the world outside.

I began to write this book at a time when I was trying to come to terms with loss—loss of old relationships, old homes, loss of my past from moving on and growing older. I had become aware that the important landscapes of my past were no longer there when I returned to find them. I felt a great discrepancy between what I remembered and what I saw when I went again to an old haunt and found it changed, went again to see an old lover and found her remote. My images of my past, of a scene as it was when I left it or first lived it, were so vivid in my mind that the incongruities between what I remembered and what I saw outside myself disturbed me.

I decided I did not want to lose the images that were once so important to me. I would write about them and thus hold on to those landscapes that had lasting meaning. I began writing about "things no longer there" in a deliberately pictorial way, painting my inner pictures to stem the tides of change. This volume represents that painting; though verbal, the sense of it is highly pictorial. I speak of the glow of a desert at dawn, of the quietness of a coastside marsh, of the remembered chatter of girls splashing in a lake in a summer camp, of the daily rituals of a lesbian intimacy.

I speak, too, of the experience of losing my eyesight. Not long after I had begun work on this book, I started to lose vision in both my eyes. Objects I previously saw in the outer world were now no longer visible to me. This experience seemed very much in keeping with my theme of disappearing external landscapes. Most importantly, my loss of sight focused my attention on the value of inner vision, those inner images that so brilliantly organize the world and that are made up of much more than visual clues, but persist through their emotional meanings.

The guiding theme of *Things No Longer There* is the struggle to honor inner images, the important ones to each of us, especially when the outer world changes, seeming to obliterate what once was so central. Each chapter explores this theme in a different setting. Together they offer a mosaic of memories and visions, moving back and forth in time. Part I contains stories about my returning to geographic landscapes of my past and finding them no longer as they once were. Facing such loss, I create images of the invisible physical landscapes that were once so meaningful to me. In Part II, I explore invisible lesbian landscapes, often hidden beneath the veneer of the heterosexual world, to highlight important aspects of lesbian social realities. In Part III, on blindness and sight, I describe my experiences while losing my eyesight. I share my internal world to reveal processes of readjustment and reorientation to a world felt when not seen, to a world known through inner and constantly changing vision. In a final, novella-length story presented in Part IV, I take the reader back to a time in my life when one particular personal relationship assumed great importance for me. I render that relationship here as a poignant intimate drama. Each section of the book mixes stories of searching, whether for lost geographic landscapes or invisible emotional landscapes, stories of recovering past visions that stand as testimony to the compelling power of inner portraits.

Things No Longer There: A Memoir of Losing Sight and Finding Vision is intended both for the general reader and as a contribution to the academic fields of qualitative sociology, feminist ethnography, and lesbian and disability studies. This book extends a method I previously articulated in *Social Science and the Self: Personal Essays on an Art Form* (1991), in which I argued for the value of a subjective approach to the development of knowledge. It further elaborates themes concerning gender and identity I addressed in my studies *The Mirror Dance: Identity in a Women's Community* (1983) and *The Family Silver: Essays on Relationships among Women* (1996).

Like my earlier works, *Things No Longer There* experiments with narrative form. It provides a unique journey both personally inward and outward to various parts of the country. It is a travelogue, a set of inner portraits painted with a loving hand, a glimmer of hope, a set of words and images thrown up against loss. As I wrote each chapter, I felt I was gaining self-acceptance from valuing my inner visions, and I enjoyed the activity of writing as if I was painting.

Now I invite the reader to come with me as I go birdwatching before sunrise, as I drive down the California coast, as I look for lesbians at a folk music festival, as I learn to walk with a white cane. Come with me as I look for an old love. Let my memories spark yours. Let my visions encourage your own internal pictures, for this is a book about valuing inner vision and about unusual kinds of sight. I hope it enriches the life of the reader by stimulating meaningful emotions and insights that will last well beyond the reading.

PART I

Vanishing Landscapes

ONE

Things No Longer There

I TEND TO GIVE exact directions. A friend, noticing this once, told me about how her father gave directions: "You turn left at the corner where the big tree used to be in front of that house they tore down last year, then right in a few blocks where the pharmacy was, near the stoplight." The image of trees and buildings no longer standing in the midwestern town where my friend grew up, but that were still very present in her father's mind, has stayed with me for a long time, those absent features of the landscape more visible to me than many places I have seen. Perhaps that is because the missing elements were the only ones my friend told me about and because they had a compelling hold on her father's imagination, but more likely because I, too, am drawn to places no longer there, to imagined scenes, wished for experiences, to sad, sad feelings of longing for things past that never really occurred exactly as I have remembered them.

A few years ago, I had a strange experience concerning my past that raised confusing questions for me. I was back East visiting my family. My sister suggested we drive out into the country to look for a summer camp we once went to, so one morning, seven of us piled into her station wagon—my sister and her husband, my lover and myself, and my sister's three girls. We drove out to the river valley area where the camp was located and up into the surrounding hills, taking winding roads that seemed familiar but whose names we did not know. We were wandering around looking for the camp and for the small lake on which it was built. The camp had been at one end of the lake, its center a large grassy field that sloped down to the water's edge. Off to one side of the lake, back in the woods, were cabins for campers; on the opposite side was a pioneer unit made of tents. A T-shaped wooden pier extended out into the water at the base of the grassy field. Counselors walked on this pier supervising girls in different swimming groups in the water. Rowboats and canoes were docked nearby, but the main impression was of the lake— a calm expanse of quiet, dark water surrounded on all sides, except where the camp was, by dense brush and high trees. The woods on the far sides of the lake were occupied by no one and felt like a wilderness. Counselors and campers never took trips into those woods for fear of getting lost, or perhaps because someone else owned that land.

I went to this camp as a camper for one year at age fourteen. The next year, I was a counselor in training, and the next year, a counselor. I liked the camp, a girls' camp, because it was tightly run and because I could do outdoor athletic activities and, very importantly, contradictory as it sounds, be freed of the constraints of being a girl—of feeling less good than others, more awkward, more internal, and less well liked. At the camp, I could be adventuresome, wild, individual, brush my hair back, get tan and dirty, run fast, pull pranks, and fall in love with the camp director and certain other counselors and campers. I always wanted to be like those others who were more naturally athletic and aloof than I was. I wanted others to like me, and fortunately I felt that I was viewed with affection at the camp. During my summers there, I got a chance to be good at things, while the rest of the year, at school, I was second best to boys. I often wondered what I would do when I was back at school again. I had images of myself standing at a free-throw line shooting eighty baskets in a row. I did not play basketball, but I wanted to do something that would show I was someone special, as I had felt during my summers at the camp.

One entered the camp grounds on a dirt road that led in from the paved county road. A large, brown wooden building on stilts—the dining hall—stood immediately to one side upon entering. Across the way, a low-lying white farmhouse, with a broad open porch, looked out over the lake. Surrounding it was the large grassy field, and next to it a black-topped tennis court, which was important to me because tennis was my main activity at the time, my main way of proving myself. The farmhouse contained the camp infirmary and was the summer home of the camp director and another woman who co-owned the camp with her. These two women were a lesbian couple, but I did not know that then. I doubt that the parents of the eighty girls who attended the camp each month of the summer would have left their daughters there had they known.

We knew them as "Miss Sandy" and "Mrs. Sullivan," two women from New Jersey who sometimes took trips to Europe together and owned this camp. Mrs. Sullivan was quiet, older, stayed in the background, and had a halo of thick, short, gray hair. She arrived at the camp each summer several weeks later than Miss Sandy, as if to make clear that she came from a different place and a different life. She had several grown children, played the cello in a symphony, and had a bedroom upstairs in the white farmhouse. Miss Sandy, the camp director, had a spacious room downstairs with a single bed in it that never seemed used for sleep. Papers and supplies were always laid out on it.

Miss Sandy's real name was Jeannette Marion, but no one called her that. She had sandy hair—from which she got her nickname—a wiry, compact body, and muscular legs. She ran the camp with much intensity and as if she knew everything about everyone. Occasionally, she told us about the men she had once dated, but more often about how she had been a gym teacher in New Jersey and, for a long time, had a dream of owning a girls' camp. She had saved her money constantly until she and Mrs. Sullivan found this camp. They named it Camp Tyrolé after a trip they once took to the Tyroléan Alps in Austria. Their story of that trip always dutifully included the fact that another woman was along with them and that Mrs. Sullivan joined Miss Sandy over there later. Camp Tyrolé was Miss Sandy's dream come true. She ran it based on a philosophy of individual needs. Each day, she decided which activities to schedule and assigned each counselor her duties. She let the campers pick their activities after each meal—archery, horseback riding, tennis, swimming. Sitting at our long tables in the dining hall, we raised our hands to say what we wanted and Miss Sandy counted hands and noticed who got what.

Now, twenty-eight years after having last been there, my sister and I were wandering around looking for Miss Sandy's camp. I mentioned to my sister that I thought Mrs. Sullivan and Miss Sandy were probably a lesbian couple, but lesbianism is not a subject we discuss. I thought Miss Sandy had probably died by now; Mrs. Sullivan most definitely had. It was too late to visit and tell them that I, too, was a lesbian and that it had been a great camp. I had learned psychology there at the many staff meetings in the evenings when Miss Sandy led discussions of the emotional well-being of each camper.

We drove around for some time looking for the camp and not finding it. At one point, I saw an opening in the woods beside the road that looked like the place where the pioneer unit had been. A large granite rock sitting behind a pink ranch-style house seemed like the spot where the pioneer unit campers had once launched their canoes out onto the lake. My sister and I thought of going out and looking more closely to see if this really was the place, but I worried, what if someone came out of the house and asked what we were doing there? What if dogs barked at us? My sister's husband stopped the car and I looked for a long time at a clearing near the house where the bushes seemed familiar. I remembered the interior of the only tent in the pioneer unit I had ever been in.

We got out of the car farther away around a bend where the road was less inhabited and a muddy path led into the woods behind parked construction equipment. Trailing three children and two adults, my sister and I walked in on this path intent on finding the lake, only to find that the path ended near a pile of building supplies. Workmen, who were standing around, said there was a lake in the distance, but I could not see it. I thought I saw edges of buildings that may have been campers' cabins. Walking back to the car, I stared at a small, brown shacklike house we had passed on the way in. It looked like one of the cabins from the camp now added onto and inhabited. Cans with flowers in them were set out on both sides of the front door.

We got back in the car, headed quickly around in a big circle, and stopped where a driveway turnoff may have been the old road leading to the camp. As we drove in on this road, I saw a red house on stilts to the side up a slight hill. Someone came out on the front deck of the house to watch us. Across the way, where the white farmhouse had been, there was now a peach-colored house that stood two stories high and dominated the landscape. A basketball hoop hung above a garage door in front of the house and a broad cement driveway spread forward toward us in all directions. Dobermans came out to greet us. Two young boys, who had been playing outside, came over to talk with us after we had stepped out of the car and were walking around. Then their father came out. We asked after the camp. He did not know of one, but then he thought maybe he had heard of it. His wife came out and began puttering in the background.

I had a hard time seeing the lake. It was in the distance behind the house, but it looked a lot smaller and farther away than I had remembered it. It did not really look much like a lake. Then I finally thought I saw—down near the edge, where the lake used to meet the shore—an overgrowth of bushes that may have hid a path that had once led down to the younger campers' cabins. It was just past where the Arts and Crafts building had been. I asked my sister if those bushes looked to her like where the path had been, pointing in the direction of the mound of brush. We asked the father if there was a path down there, and if there were cabins in the woods. He said he had never been back there and that his boys did not go back beyond that point. The brush was too thick.

I had never before had such a feeling of erasure. We were not in a girls' camp but in a nest of residences. I wondered what had happened to my past. I thought I must be getting old since I wanted so much to see the past and not the present. I could not put two and two together. How could the camp be gone? How could these houses be here? Had these people no respect? What had they done to the lake? Where was Miss Sandy? I even missed the old black-topped tennis court. We had come too late. What would we say to my sister's girls—"This used to be our camp"? How could something as definite as the large grassy field and the farmhouse and the big brass bell on the front porch that Miss Sandy used to ring to wake us all up be gone? How could it have become so invisible? Was this what would happen to the rest of my life?

When I think of that day, I see pink and orange houses and spots of bushes that look familiar. I felt confused, as if I had lost my inner bearings, although it was the outer world that had changed. I did not like what I saw. We got back into the car and drove out past the red house on stilts. I was sure that house had been the dining hall. I was sure this was where the camp had been. My sister and I reassured each other. We had found it.

We drove back along the river valley the way we had come and had lunch in a diner in an old industrial town by the side of the river. That diner had always been there, even back at the time of the camp. I wondered why the diner was still there when the camp was gone. Why was it not also someone's house? Why wasn't it leveled? Was there something about a girls' camp, a woman's dream, two lesbians who no one knew were lesbian, who invented self-protective stories and had schedules that showed them as unconnected, and who helped each other fulfill their dreams? Was there something about what was erased that mattered, and what I was attached to? Was I destined to be among the invisible? How hard that seems to me. Did it matter that the camp was no longer there? It was there when it counted, for Miss Sandy and for me and my sister. I once nailed a xylophone onto the top of the seat of Miss Sandy's dining hall chair, hiding it beneath the cushion she sat on. She made me take it off and she did not think it was funny. Only later did I realize that I had never hammered anything onto either of my parents' chairs and that I had felt I needed to prove my presence.

My sister had wanted us to go back and see. I went in search of the camp not because I thought I needed to go, but to please my sister and because it was something we could do, that day, with the children. I think my sister often tries to recreate her childhood, but in ways that make it better. She was one of three children and she has three children and she often does things with them that remind her of what she liked when she was a girl. I fear recreating my past, but I have a similar need. Yet it is not the past of a family I seek so much as of intimate relationships that will hold me and give me something I did not have before, or that I had only a promise of.

I will long remember that day when my sister and I went back to the place where our camp used to be and found it no longer there. By the time we left, I had seen myself again in splashes of water out on a lake near a pier listening to the giggles of many small frolicking girls, in a moment of adolescent self-consciousness when I sat outside the dining hall near the dusty entry road and worried about whether others in a summer camp would like me. I think there is no telling how often we see what is not there, how often we mourn our losses in order to feel our gains. Time, or what happens in time, seems to turn my life into inner pictures that are more present, more real, more everything life is supposed to be than back when an experience was external and new. Amidst the square-shaped modern homes, I saw again the low white farmhouse, the lawn sloping down to the lake, Miss Sandy, wearing khaki shorts, coming outside behind the farmhouse to talk to me. I was shy and looked at the ground and tears came to my eyes when I spoke. The camp, the scene is gone now, but I see it clearly.

TWO

The Vision Fire

When I first witnessed the effects of the Vision Fire in 1996, I was not aware that I was beginning to lose my eyesight. While I never again would see Point Reyes as clearly as I had in the months right after a wildfire altered the landscape, I would keep my sense of delight in that earlier experience, which has become a lasting inner vision for me.

LAST YEAR, POINT REYES BURNED. The 90,000 acre national seashore that juts out into the Pacific like a bent elbow north of San Francisco burned in a huge fire that lasted for sixteen days. The fire started near the summit of a hill near Tomales Bay and burned all the way to the sea, sending up massive dark clouds of smoke, raging over hillsides through dense green brush and trees, incinerating everything in its path. It devoured a central area of the park measuring five miles long by as wide. It was a cloud-shaped burn that narrowed toward the ridges from which the fire came. When it was through, the broad hills facing the ocean were covered with gray cinder and ash, with white ash on top that looked like snow. Scorched, blackened tree trunks stood occasionally in bare spaces, their branches broken off, reminders of all the rest that had burned.

I had been planning to go to Point Reyes the very week the fire started. I wanted to go to the beach with my lover to celebrate our anniversary. It was a time of crisp, cool autumn days. I wanted to see the birds start to migrate. Then I heard that Point Reyes was on fire and we did not go. A month later, we went to a section of the park that had escaped the fire. On the way, we stopped for groceries in a small town near where the fire began and I smelled the burn in the air. It was a damp, dark, ashy, musky smell. We continued on, since I did not want to go into the burned area, to be disturbed by seeing the destruction. After that, I stayed away from Point Reyes for six months. I heard reports about the fire—that the four boys who had started it had turned themselves in, that some areas of the park were closed, that two weeks after the fire was over, new green growth was poking up through the gray ash, nourished by the winter rains.

I finally went again to Point Reyes in the beginning of May. At that time, my lover and I decided to drive the fire route to the sea. We turned off onto a road leading through the center of the fire area, which had been closed down for months because the fire had crossed it, jumped a few houses, and marched on. As it marched, I was told, the animals took flight, some of them swimming when they reached the inlets and ponds near the ocean. They say the deer swam and the small foxes, too. As we drove, at first things looked as they had before the fire. On both sides of the road was thick, gray-green brush and tall trees. Then occasional singed trees and branches started to appear. The road carved a tunnel through the dense brush and wound upward. As we neared the top of a hill, it suddenly felt open and bright. Thin blades of fresh grass were shooting up in the dappled sunlight all around us. Amidst the grass, charred, blackened poles that had once been trees were climbing the hillside. They stood as if marching up the hill, guarding the fire area, welcoming us in. The stark beauty of those dark trees set against the new, green grass surprised me. I had expected grayness and depressing feelings.

Instead, I was seeing sparkling, delicate, fresh, white-green growth and the silhouetted black trees.

As we drove further, the view opened out to an expanse of bright-green hillsides sprawling for miles, dotted here and there with groups of burnt tree trunks; the blue ocean was in the distance, the road winding toward it. The road soon became lined with tall, yellow wildflowers tossing about in the wind and sun. Several times, I saw nearby a charred, black tree that seemed still intact, its curved branches held high in a rounded canopy on top, yet the whole thing black and leafless, its sculpted dark outlines suggesting the life that had once been here. These rounded black trees seemed more beautiful to me than any live tree. I felt as if I was in an artwork.

After driving through the broad hills, we descended toward the ocean and arrived at the place where the road ends and the sky meets the sea. Ahead, the marshes and estuaries spread out like large glassy, flat puddles in a muddy basin, the beach lying behind them. Walking toward the beach, I passed a marsh area where I saw many black skeletons of bushes with round shapes that looked like small versions of the larger burnt trees. Then standing on the glistening beach, I looked back at the hills we had just come across. They sloped down toward the ocean and were bare but for a covering of new green growth and a few burnt trees. I felt I could see every blade of grass. Things were so very clear. I had been wrong, I thought. The fire, the devastation, was not bad but good, invigorating, a fresh start, a new canvas on which had been painted only the brightest colors. It was a painting full of fresh green in which someone had dabbed in a few dark trees. There were only the clearest outlines, the truest, basic silhouettes.

I later learned that the new growth was so vivid in color because the winter rains had been plentiful, and because—as a result of the fire—all the old, dense brush that had kept out the sunlight was now gone, so grasses and flowers that had not seen much light for years were growing and thriving. These were indeed the bare essentials, the delicate new statement, "I am here," these thin grasses that had not weathered storms before.

As I stood on the beach that day looking back at the green hills, I felt I, too, had a new lease on life. Had I known before how beautiful it would be, I would not have been afraid to come to the burnt area of Point Reyes. How fascinating it would have been to have seen every inch of the new growth, the change, the coloring that came after the devastation. Now I wished I had come earlier. Even more importantly, my experience that day made me believe in art. I felt that no photograph could truly capture it, no real vision could be this clear, this unreal. We left the beach after a while, but my view looking back from it at the newly green hills stays in my mind. I have thought a lot about why that particular artwork appealed to me—the spareness, the clear lines, the fresh new colors, the Japanese aesthetic. Nothing was crowded; there were spaces between things; objects stood out. It was like the desert—big shapes, big expanses— but green. It was a large, complete challenge to the senses; no vision was impaired.

I visited Point Reyes several more times that spring and summer. Each time, I marveled at the landscape. As the summer wore on, the colors toned down and my sense of the absolute newness of things faded. But as more wildflowers bloomed, the changes continued and the place still felt special to me. Then in mid-July, hoping for explanations—wanting to learn more about the new growth I was seeing—I went with my lover on a naturalist-led walk through part of the fire area. The walk was scheduled to start in a dirt parking lot near a ridge trail with scenic views toward the ocean. We arrived early and waited. Soon a white van pulled up. Out of it stepped a woman park ranger wearing a brown uniform and a black backpack. As she turned away, I saw on the very top-center of her pack a small rainbow insignia. Ranger Maureen was a lesbian, or so I thought, although no one ever mentioned that fact, just as no one ever mentioned that my lover and I were a lesbian couple.

19

Another car pulled up and a woman got out wearing shorts and carrying a baby. She talked with Ranger Maureen as if they were old friends. This second woman later referred to her husband, settling the question of whether or not she was a lesbian—to the extent that question ever does get settled. She had worked for the Park Service as a firefighter at first, until she was injured, and now she managed crews restoring portions of the burnt area of the park. Although this was her day off, she had come for the fire walk and to help Ranger Maureen.

Next to arrive were twelve to fifteen teenagers, who walked in out of the woods wearing dusty tee shirts and jeans and carrying shovels. They were a crew of summer Youth Conservation Corps workers who were clearing the trails in the park in the aftermath of the fire and pulling out invasive non-native plants. They were going on this walk to learn more about effects of the fire and the regrowth. A few other women drove up and soon all of us were standing around in a big circle in the dusty parking lot, surrounded on all sides by burnt and unburnt trees, and Ranger Maureen was taking out photographs, passing them around and telling us about her experiences during the fire.

She said that the fire had been exciting and she spoke of it as something good, which surprised me. I felt it was bad and that she was putting a good face on it, justifying it because it had occurred. Then she told us that the trees all around us were Bishop pines and that it took a fire to release the seeds from their cones, which then fell to the ground and germinated to start new growth. The Point Reyes' current Bishop pine forest was old, she said. The big trees we were surrounded by would soon die. These Bishop pines seemed to me unusually graceful trees, their branches lifted upward like bent arms raised. If we looked closely at the ground, the ranger said, we would see the new small Bishop pine sprouts. They were only three to six inches tall. Only some of them would survive. They would become the new forest of Bishop pines that would last for the next century. I looked down at the ground at a few of the small pine shoots near me and then off into the distance at the green hills that stretched toward the ocean. I would not be alive to see the new forest, I thought. It would take a long time.

The fire turned everything gray, Ranger Maureen told us as she passed around photographs showing the area covered with gray ash, with the snow-white ash on top of it. Each photograph was mounted on a piece of cardboard and had a plastic covering on top of it to protect it from grimy hands. "No one knew what to do with a fire that big. They didn't know how to put it out," she said. "It burned its way out by going to the sea. The animals fled out in front of it. The bulldozers didn't know how to follow the trails."

"We had trouble with the 'dozers," the woman with the baby joined in. "They couldn't find the fire roads that were right there. They bulldozed in places they shouldn't have. The Park Service people had trouble telling the firefighters what to do. Anyone see the 'dozers?" she asked the kids, who murmured back unintelligibly.

Ranger Maureen explained why the fire was exciting: things burned, but you did not usually get to see them close up. "We had kept the park from getting burned by protecting it for many years," she said. "During the fire, people were calling in with more questions than we could answer. I was on the phones. It was exciting to watch it. We didn't know what would happen next." She told us she had been coming to this Bay View Trail almost every day since the fire. Right after the fire, the whole area was gray; she could not imagine things would grow back. She had watched the new growth inch by inch. The first thing that came back was the fiddlehead fern. They had a root system underground that enabled them to survive the heat of the fire above the ground. At first, there was nothing, she said. Then two days after the fire, amazingly, the ferns started poking their heads up. The ash had trapped the dampness. Then the fern heads started unfolding. It was wonderful to see them.

We began to walk out along the trail, Ranger Maureen pointing out fiddlehead ferns by the side of the trail and the many Bishop pine sprouts that were shooting up—tiny spikes only a few inches tall. The trail we were walking on was actually a dirt path wide enough for a vehicle. "When the trees and shrub burned away," Ranger Maureen explained, gesturing broadly with her hand, "the birds and small animals had no place to hide. The hawks and other predators had a field day. They could see their prey clearly." She pointed to an upturned root system by the side of the trail that had belonged to a tree now burned away. New plants had started growing opportunistically within the roots and dirt, taking advantage of the moisture. She pointed to the poison oak that was coming back everywhere. This area looked very different at first, she said. What we were seeing now was actually the second generation of new growth. Some plants that grew very quickly at first were now gone, or they were being squeezed out by the newer plant growth. Can anyone figure out why? she asked the group and waited patiently for answers, like a good teacher. People suggested that the first wave of plants were eaten, or that the root systems of the older plants were big and strong, and although they took time to regrow, they produced a lot of growth when they did return.

As we walked on, everything seemed to glow. Small, fresh green leaves glowed on the hillsides across the way; even the burnt, brown tree trunks glowed darkly in the sun. Both the leaves and the skeletal outlines of the trees seemed clearly defined in the soft light. Beyond these closer hills, the estuaries and ponds out near the ocean shimmered like mirrors. Out in that direction was the beach where I had walked with my lover a couple of months before. The rolling hills that had burned and were now bright green extended broadly toward the ocean. Here and there they were cut through as if decorated with tan ribbons—the dirt fire roads and trails that curved over the hills. When the brush and trees had burned away, these paths were exposed so that now they were all visible. With one giant step, I felt, I might land on one of the trails and walk on it, striding across the hills. In a few steps, I would be at the ocean. But, in fact, the trails ran for miles.

The woman with the baby, who now carried her child high on her back, told us that after the fire many things that could not be seen before became visible. One man she knew found a red bicycle of his that had been stolen when he was six. It was discovered when the brush burned away, exposing an old dump that had been completely grown over. When they found it, he said, "That's my bike." He was now a grown man with a kid of his own, but he knew it was his bike. People were finding things.

Our group of about two dozen was straggling by now—the kids in their baggy jeans, a few other women in shorts, my lover and myself, and the two leaders. Ranger Maureen pointed to a large hill and peak in front of us, called Mount Vision, where the fire started. Because it started there, the Forest Service and the local people called it the Vision Fire. I thought the name was appropriate, because the fire revealed things, both new and old. Ranger Maureen soon began to discuss poison oak, which I thought was probably a common subject of outdoor people. She said she ate small amounts of it regularly—to get immune to it, or to decrease its effects when she touched it. The woman with the baby said she had tried to eat it too, but her throat swelled and she had to be hospitalized. The kids, darting out from the group occasionally to pull up invasive plants by the trailside, looked suspiciously at the poison oak nearby as if it would eat them.

In a sunny area in the shadow of Mount Vision, we finally reached a clearing. "We'll come to the burnt foundations of some homes," Ranger Maureen said. "We'll stop there. Take a look around. People really shouldn't build their houses so close to trees." Her implication was that this was why the houses burned. The kids scattered quickly into a gray, cindery foundation near the trail where once a house had stood. The foundation was square-shaped and edged by burnt, blackened wood planks. People started picking up small pieces of burnt metal and china. I saw a white saucer and a blue vase that were still intact. They sat there in the sun and seemed so misplaced without the house that had once surrounded them. On a hillside across the way, two other houses that had not completely burned were being rebuilt; their redwood decks looked fresh. But nothing grew here on this gray ash and cinder base that looked so small. I thought that the other houses should have burned too. No one should build a house in a national park. I felt the heat of the sun. The Conservation Corps crew soon began disappearing down a path on the other side of the burnt foundation. They were heading downhill toward a parking area where the cars and trucks they had come in on were waiting for them.

With the kids gone, that left only the ranger, the woman with the baby, three other women, my lover, and myself. Our return walk along the trail was more intimate and more relaxed than the walk out. The talk was more personal, more gossipy. I learned that Ranger Maureen, young as she looked, had a small daughter, and I wondered if she had been married, or if she was a single lesbian mother. I suspected the latter, perhaps because I wanted it that way. I wondered if she had a lover. But the talk never got that intimate. Indeed, I never really knew for certain that Ranger Maureen was a lesbian. It was something I just felt.

After a while, the woman with the baby turned to Ranger Maureen, who was walking beside her, and said, "The four boys who started the fire were on the walk." The silence was thick and sudden. I was stunned, and I felt deeply touched. I wondered which ones they were. Was one of them that small boy who kept going off to the side of the trail by himself and sitting there, seeming not to fit in, not quite the outdoorsy, nature type? He wore a gold chain around his neck and baggy pants; he was just a young kid, nervous and watchful. I thought, why did it matter to me to know who the boys were?

Ranger Maureen caught her breath. "I hadn't known," she said. "I hope I didn't say anything that upset them." She remembered she had said that the fire destroyed people's homes. I remembered she had said that animals died. But I felt she had emphasized the good things. Anyone who had set that fire would have been pleased to have been on the walk. I felt that being in the Conservation Corps crew working to restore the fire area probably helped the kids. It was a terrible thing to have on your conscience burning down a national park.

"Having the boys work to clear the trails was part of the community's healing process," the woman with the baby said. "The boys' parents and the community decided on it as their community service."

"They're good kids," she added. "They turned themselves in. The father of one of the boys is a fire fighter himself, so he knew how to put out a fire. He thought they had put out their fire that night, but they hadn't and it went underground. From where the fire started, we knew it had to be local kids. When I was a kid, I lived around here and we used to go to that same spot to get away from our parents. It's a teenage hangout back there. You climb up to it from behind the houses."

As I listened, I thought, but it was an illegal place to make a fire. It was illegal to make a fire at all at that time.

"We would sneak out at night and go off and spend time in the woods," the woman with the baby said.

I could see them in my mind as she spoke, four boys sitting around under the trees at dusk and in the evening, making a fire—four boys not quite old enough, talking to each other in monosyllables. I then thought about how California it was, this story about kids who had burnt down a national wilderness area and then were being reclaimed by doing something that was good for them. The boy I thought was one of them had looked like he felt pretty miserable as he sat beside the trail. Maybe he wasn't one of them at all, just a kid tired from the afternoon sun and from pulling plants. I asked the woman with the baby which ones the boys were, but she said she would not tell, implying I ought not to have asked. Only she knew they would be on our walk and she had come along for that reason. I thought about women keeping secrets and watching out for kids. Such watching out for the kids who had threatened the park, like the watching out for the park itself, seemed congruent. This place was so watched out for that the fire was viewed not as a catastrophe but as a chance to see things usually not seen—to find an old bicycle, to see the regrowth; it was a chance for my lover and me to experience a special place, a chance for me to feel I had found something quite my own.

We arrived back in the dusty parking lot beneath the Bishop pines, where we had started out just a couple of hours earlier. It seemed odd to me how my experience had changed. At first, it was about a landscape that burned and turned gray and then became bright green, and all of a sudden it was about four boys and doing right by them. I had met a woman forest ranger; certainly the dream of many lesbian girls is to become a forest ranger, if not a cowboy. I had often wanted to be a forest ranger myself. On the nature walk, my images had changed over time from scenery to people. I was glad I had gone. I was also glad that my lover and I had our own private walk and drive through the fire area earlier. I think I liked best the fresh, bare, new feeling of the landscape after the fire. Often, I like to feel that things are fresh and new—as when I am alone; or when I write something new; or when I am with another woman and what is between us seems as if it has never happened anywhere else in just this way.

When the old is stripped away, the new growth can be seen. That was one of the lessons of the fire for me. The fire made me appreciate what I could see. It made me feel I needed defined spaces and a sense of clarity and protectedness. I liked how Ranger Maureen had called this wilderness area and seashore a park. To me, that meant it was a special, cared-for place that people could visit and appreciate, that I could enjoy without feeling as if I was trespassing.

On my first trip to Point Reyes after the fire, when I had walked on the beach and looked back at the startlingly green hillside, I had wanted to take a photograph. But no picture could capture what I was seeing. Often when I take a photograph, the result pales compared with my mental image. I blame it on the camera when the true problem is a discrepancy between my inner image and what lies outside, or what is taken in by some other means. The task for me always seems to lie in the process of inventing, of creating a protected, aesthetically pleasing world where I can find comfort. That invented inner world is my photograph, my image. I think there was *the* fire and there is *my* fire, and that mine is an artwork quite rarely seen in nature. But occasionally nature provides a basis for my image—an outline, a sense of light or color that feels very much mine.

The Point Reyes fire, called by locals and by the national seashore staff the Vision Fire, started on October 3, 1995, near the summit of a hill called Mount Vision and burned to the sea. I visited Point Reyes during the spring and summer after the fire. A year later, I went back again in the spring. By then, the trees that had once been black and clearly silhouetted like dark sticks against the green hills were bleached white or turning gray. They were weathering. Scrub had grown back on the hillsides, in the ravines, and near the inlets by the sea. The whole view was softer. Things blended in. The sense of extreme clarity and definition that so pleased me and that had marked the aftermath of the fire was now gone.

THREE

Saving a Tree

No sooner had I begun exploring the theme of "things no longer there" than I began seeing examples of it everywhere. I wrote this backyard story when I woke one morning to find the geography of my daily landscape changing. Though the story is about saving a tree, it is also about saving one's own inner memories.

IN THE YARD BEHIND MY HOUSE is a big, misshapen Monterey pine towering high above all the houses nearby. The tree's upper limbs are green and reach toward the blue sky. But the gray lower limbs and trunk are shorn and bare, as if someone took a chain saw and sliced off all the growth further down, leaving only that bright green canopy on top, which is in fact what happened. Several months ago, some men came out—those hired hands, hired guns—and they started to chop the tree down. I woke that morning to the sound of a snarling saw. I looked out my bedroom window and saw nothing. Then I heard the saw grinding loudly and continuously. I called my neighbor, a woman who is a gardener and knows trees. "We'd better go," she said. "They can cut down a tree in twenty minutes."

I met her out front and we went around the block. There, in the rear of an overgrown lot, a square-chested man with a broad leather belt around his waist and a bright-orange chain saw in his hand stood holding the saw above his head against the gray trunk of the tree. He had already cut off three lower limbs.

"Stop," I said.

"Can't," he answered, holding the saw poised, ready to strike again. "This tree's going to come down."

"Who hired you?" I asked.

"I can't tell you that."

"We like this tree. I want to call whoever hired you. Maybe you can just trim it."

"No time," he said. "I have to get this job done." He looked around at the three other men in his crew, who were already hauling off branches. "I've got to eat," he said.

I was shocked as much by his rationale as by the tree coming down. How could I argue with a man's right to eat, or with a chain saw? I felt like all the radical environmentalists I had ever heard of, who might lay down their lives to protect an endangered species. He pulled the cord on the orange saw once again, turning it on. I saw myself going up to the tree trunk, standing between it and the man with the orange saw and its three-foot extended blade, daring him to cut. But I stood still, at a distance from the tree, and instead, I started talking. I started carrying on like a woman facing a man with a gun, a brick wall, an inexorable force, an army marching to war. I felt quite hysterical and I did not like the feeling. I did not want to be an impulsive woman facing a recalcitrant and bullying man, matching him word for word, sentiment for sentiment.

"I'm going to cut," he said.

"No, you're not."

He raised the saw up in the direction of a lower limb.

"You're really tough. You're just a big man with a saw."

"You don't know what you're talking about."

"Neither do you. The neighbors like this tree. It protects us."

29

"I've got another job this afternoon. I don't have time for this."

"Do you get pleasure out of cutting down trees?"

"Why don't you go home?"

"I am home."

"It's legal," he said.

By this time, my neighbor had visited an adjacent house and found out the name of the contractor and of the owner of the lot.

"I know who hired you," I said. "I'm going to call the owner. Stop cutting while I call."

"I'll give you twenty minutes."

"Half an hour, and I don't want to hear that saw. I'll be right back if I hear that saw."

"Fuck you," he muttered loud enough for me to hear.

"You too," I called back.

He lowered the orange saw with its long, chain-linked blade and laid it on the ground.

I walked quickly back around the block with my neighbor. At home, I called the contractor and the owner. The owner turned out to be an elderly couple who lived near Sacramento, but who used to live around here when this area was mostly ranchland and a stream ran down the middle of our street. I spoke first with the woman. She told me she had planted the tree a long time ago. She never expected it to grow that big. Now a neighbor had complained. Branches had grown near his house, which stood next to the tree. The woman and her husband feared what it would cost if the tree did damage to the neighbor's house. If she had known the tree would get that large, she never would have planted it so close to houses, she said. It was not the kind of tree you plant near a house.

Then she told me she had not seen the tree in years, but she and her husband figured it was cheaper to cut it down than to trim it. The trimming would just have to be done again. They were planning to sell the property soon. People would not buy it with a big tree like that in back. Or if they did, they'd just cut the tree down.

She sounded pained, as if this headache of a tree so far away was not what she wanted.

"We will lose money if we only cut it back," she finally said. "The dumpster had to be pre-paid. We had to get a big one to haul off all the debris." I was struck with how quickly the tree had become debris.

She paused, then she put her husband on. "No," he told me repeatedly. "I'm not going to change my mind. You don't understand. The ground there is weak; it's marshy there. The tree could fall over at any time." He then began to lecture me on what the neighborhood used to be like when he lived here and the stream out in front had to be crossed by a bridge. "All this land is wet," he said. "It's unstable."

"The stream in the yards changed its course years ago," I told him. "We're not unstable. We're on bedrock." I then accused him of insensitivity to trees and of being an out-of-touch absentee landlord, arguing with him as I had with the man with the orange saw. I was surprised by my willingness to badger an elderly man. I finally asked my lover, Hannah, to speak with him. He also told her no. "He won't budge," she said after hanging up. My neighbor, a sweet, soft-spoken woman, then called him. "He said no," she reported, seeming dejected, forlorn.

The contractor soon arrived. I opened my front door to a small, neatly dressed, wiry, smooth-talking man who acted conciliatory and spoke of our options. He sat in our living room talking with the three of us. If we let them cut the tree down, he said, he would plant us four birch saplings out near our back fence instead. All we would have to do was water them. Or the tree could stay up and be trimmed and he would give us the saplings anyway. The offer sounded odd to me. But Hannah and my neighbor seriously considered it, which frightened me. How could they not see the smoke-screen? I wondered.

I acted friendly and was cordial with the contractor. I wanted to make up for having acted so badly in arguing with the tree cutter and the elderly owner. I told the contractor the tree protected us from the noisy street behind it; the neighbors in the yards all liked that tree. No one had asked us about it. The tree was trimmed five years ago with no problem.

"Wasn't there another woman?" he asked me. "Over with my men? You're too nice to be her."

"I am her," I said. "Your man was threatening me with a chain saw."

He looked serious, and concerned.

I suddenly felt the power of my having been a hysterical woman—beyond control, making a fuss, getting in the way, calling attention to myself, being a general embarrassment. I was thinking about all the hysterical women through history—and how I had underestimated them—when the contractor's portable phone rang, jarring me. He stepped outside to answer it.

My own phone rang not long afterward. The daughter of the owners was calling. She used to live around the corner. She and I used to discuss the water from the underground stream that ran through our yard and flooded down into hers. She always used to talk to me about her sump pump.

"My parents are upset," she said.

"Can they cut the tree back?" I asked her. "The neighbors will pay for the extra cost of the dumpster."

"I'll see," she said.

Half an hour later, she called me back. "My parents will trim the tree," she said.

"How much should we make out the check for?"

"They'll pay for it."

"Are you sure?"

"They're sure."

I was surprised. I wondered why they had changed their minds. I sensed that the contractor, the parents, the daughter, and the man with the orange saw had all talked with one another on various phones.

The wiry contractor returned. He came up my front steps and knocked on the door. Standing in our living room, he talked with us briefly about how the tree should be cut. My neighbor asked him to take care with the shape of the canopy. After he left I thought about going around the block to oversee the work of the men in trimming the tree, but I did not go. A few hours later, when I went outside in my yard to look at what they had done, I saw that the tree was pretty ugly. It was painful for me to look at it. The trunk and lower limbs were bare. Raw, fleshy, round cuts reminded me of where the lower branches had once been. A bushy canopy was left on top, but it was small and it looked hollowed out. Oddly, several branches still hung down in the direction of the complaining neighbor's house. I took small comfort from the fact that the tree was still standing, straight up, planted firmly. It had certainly taken a beating. It was as if the men took their revenge by showing no care, taking no time, quickly carving off whatever they could, then leaving for the next job, the next tree, the next set of frightened neighbors.

I wished so much then that I had gone over and policed the work of those men with their saws. I would have yelled at them, "Stop. Not there. Don't you take that limb off! I will strap myself to the tree if I have to." I felt sad that I had missed that opportunity. But I had wanted not to fight anymore. I had wanted to trust that the men would do the work right.

I was told later that it is hard to save a tree. It is especially difficult when they have started cutting it down. I was told that people who want to cut down trees on their own property usually get their way. Thus, saving that tree was a triumph. What struck me most in retrospect, though, was that it was easier for me to save that tree than it is to do many other things that require a similar self-assertion—to save my job, get a better one, argue with a publisher, or tell the students in my classes what I think is true. It is harder for me, often, to answer the phone than it was to save that tree, harder to act in those more important spheres where the object is less external, the indignity more my own.

For weeks after the tree was trimmed, I could not get over how it had been mangled. When I looked out my back window, it seemed to me not the same tree it was before. Now it was imperfect. I mourned it as if it had, indeed, been cut down. Out in my yard, I tried not to look up at the hollowed-out canopy. I wished not to be reminded of what was no longer there. I wished not to be reminded of how the tree had been hurt, and of how I had failed to save it completely. I wanted to feel less exposed to the black asphalt of the street behind the tree, now visible through the spaces between the remaining limbs.

One day months later, I was out in a far back corner of my yard snipping deadheads off a rose bush when I saw a man looking up at me from a yard behind mine, next to the lot where the tree still stood. I did not recognize him.

"I'm going to build a deck," he said. "I'm clearing this yard. My partner and I are going to convert this building into condos. We'll gut it, we'll fix it up, and then we'll sell it. You know, people like the quaintness of an older building, but they really want it modern inside. I think I'll put a trellis over there."

"Don't touch that tree," I said.

"Tom and I wondered how it got to look like that," he replied. I learned that he and his partner had recently bought the house from the man who had complained about the tree.

"They were going to cut it down," I explained. Then I began to tell him the story, pleased, almost for the first time, that our tree still stood, markedly different—a tree with a story, a past, a tree that still needed us.

A few weeks later, a young woman came out to help me with some work in my yard. She was a landscape student at a city college. "I heard at school you saved a tree," she said. "Where is it?"

I pointed, smiling.

I wish I could fight all the battles, accept all the imperfections of the world around me. I wish I could hysterically throw myself in the face of whoever wants to harm me, to deny me, to stop me from growing, from standing—as that tree once did—from having all my limbs. I think that people sometimes do not understand that survival comes at a cost, that our shapes tell our stories. When I see a tree now, I wonder what its story is.

FOUR

Half Moon Bay

I wrote this story to come to terms with changes in a geographic landscape that had long been special to me. Although I began by focusing on physical changes, I soon found that my journey down the California coast took me back to the past, where inner emotional scenes were more important than changes wrought by others or by time.

LESS THEN AN HOUR FROM MY HOUSE is a town called Half Moon Bay, where a broad sweep of white-sand beach shaped like a sliver of a half moon gently embraces a cove of blue sea. When the fog lifts, the sun shines through, glinting off the glassy, blue-green water and the warm, inviting beach, producing a feeling of peacefulness. Half Moon Bay is the name of the bay and of the town, but, for me, it really means a direction, a place of mind and heart. It means a drive down along the coast to an area that is centered on Half Moon Bay but that lies mostly north and south of it. Often, I have driven a route that goes first through Pacifica, where the sky opens out over the ocean, then to Montara, that broad beach just past the rocky cliffs of Devil's Slide where cars sometimes fall to the sea and rocks sometimes fall from above, causing the road to be closed down. I pass nurseries and smell the fertilizer used on the fields of brussels sprouts and I stop only sometimes at Half Moon Bay, a town once full of farmers and old people in trailers and now full of families and professional people and condos and jumbo homes. On the main street of Half Moon Bay, more and more, are pricey shops where tourists go. I remember Half Moon Bay from a time when there was almost no downtown and no reason to stop there.

I drive farther on to San Gregorio and Pescadero, where the beaches seem to extend forever, backed by high, tan sandstone cliffs. I feel totally alone when walking the beach here in the fog, caught between the cliffs and the sea. I sometimes drive farther to Año Nuevo, a piece of shrubby overgrown land that juts out into the ocean. Elephant seals come ashore here to molt and breed and are visible farther out at sea, hanging out of the windows of a deserted house on an abandoned island. Sometimes I drive as far south as Davenport, a cement-factory town that's ashen gray beside the green sea and where an organic juice factory operates at night with eerie orange and blue lights on. It stands high on a cliff beside the sea looking out into nowhere.

I have been driving this section of the coast, walking the beaches, and visiting the forested state parks farther inland for twenty-three years now. Often I go quite regularly. I have gone on my birthday, on Thanksgiving, on weekdays and weekends, at all hours of the day and night. Even when living halfway across the country, I have come back here to visit, always feeling that when I reach the ocean, I will know what my pulse is. I will know how I feel. I will be in touch with my own inner freedom. Yet in recent years, my drive along this coast has troubled me. I have difficulty with the changes in the landscape—the new houses, the many more people. Seeing them, I feel erased, that time has passed me by, that violence has been done to me and to what is mine, or to what used to be mine. For this coast is not really mine any longer. It belongs to other people who are making it theirs.

As I drive now, I try to see the beauty of the shoreline amidst the new jumbo homes they have built on the hillsides, amidst the commuter traffic across Route 92—the one main road that links this part of the coast to the nearest inland freeway—amidst the mothers and kids playing on the once empty beaches, amidst the condos and the crowds come to see the elephant seals at Año Nuevo. I stop at San Gregorio at a coastside store and see the shaggy-haired young men hanging out at the bar, talking about the tunnel that could be built through the hills to further link this coast to civilization, talking about real estate and part-time jobs clearing lots and building houses. They talk while the country music plays on the bar stereo, and it's yesterday's country music in a revamped old country store, and the bar's on one side of a big, wood-floored room and they are listening to the Eagles' "Peaceful Easy Feeling." The nostalgia is thick here, the irony hard to miss—what's peaceful? who's easy? whose place is this?

I see the cars pulled up in the small town of Pescadero at a brown wood-shingled restaurant where it used to be only locals and beat-up hippie types came, people tired from a day at the beach, young people in jeans and full of sand who had been camping, men who had been out working coming in for morning coffee. I see the BMWs, Jaguars, and Lexuses that are now parked routinely in front of the restaurant and the women customers in jewelry and neat clothes inside sitting at the tables. The food seems much the same, though it's probably better—artichoke soup, greasy seafood (or it used to be greasy), fresh bread. I sit at the gray formica-topped counter near the kitchen, sip my soup, and try to feel again as I once did the very first time I came here—the first time I was offered artichoke soup. I look around at the people in the pine-panelled restaurant and I see, in my mind, "my coast" being gobbled up more and more each year, being overrun, and I feel I have nowhere to turn.

As I drive on, close to tears, I try to ignore these people with their new wealth, these people who I feel don't belong, who are making this area theirs and changing it in the process, who make assumptions about what they can do—that they can choose to live here, for instance, a choice I never felt I could make. It was not where my job was, it was too far away. It was part of the countryside, a place to visit, to appropriate in my fantasy—in my play life, my imagination—but not to appropriate in fact, not to build a house in, to live in permanently, not to use in that way. But that is what they've done. They have made it into a life-style choice. Each time I hear of someone who has moved to Half Moon Bay, I cringe. I feel hurt, angry, pained, and confused. I feel, "They shouldn't. It's not right. I couldn't."

On my drive now, I find I must focus through my own pain and resentment in order to see the sun glinting on the water and the roll of the hills. I focus my vision narrowly to avoid seeing the large boxy houses, the invasion of the new people. But then my own past also keeps invading, inserting itself into my vision. My trip is littered with my own inner memories as well as with the outer structures of others.

I did not always come to this coast. At first, I was afraid to come here. From where I lived inland, the ride took me over expanses of hills on winding roads. I would get dizzy and lose my bearings. Then the lush green valley and wide hills of San Gregorio would open out and I could see the sea. The first woman who took me here raised my fears. For her, the true experience of the coast was a wilderness experience and too wild for me. She always seemed to be pointing to something beyond me, something I could not do or be. When I was with her, I often felt inadequate. I felt alone and afraid and not brave enough or sturdy enough to walk the beach. But I do remember a walk on the beach at Pescadero with her in the fog once when I was not scared. That was after we parted. Only after our relationship was over was I able to feel more relaxed about this coast.

My next lover treated these beaches like home. She had been married on one of the beaches down toward Año Nuevo. I always imagined it was a hippie wedding with women in long dresses and people bringing food in baskets. She thought nothing of coming over here at night in the dark on impulse, driving the winding roads quickly through the hills. The darkness and the speed frightened me. She was the one who first took me to the restaurant in Pescadero and told me that people came for the artichoke soup and the pies. She made coming to these beaches seem normal and natural for me, like an ordinary part of life. Other people I knew back then, who worked at the bookstore where I did an hour inland, often came over to the beaches, too. When someone was missing from the bookstore because they had broken up or just were moody, they were probably out here. That bookstore group was a community. When I moved to the Midwest the next year, my mailing address, for a while, was in El Granada, a town just north of Half Moon Bay, care of a man I knew from the bookstore who lived in Menlo Park but who took his mail over here, because he had friends here.

When I drive the coast now, I am often back in those earlier times. As I near San Gregorio, I remember that some people from the bookstore later bought half the ownership in the San Gregorio Country Store, which is why it stocks lots of books. I often stop by the San Gregorio store and go in and look sideways for people I once knew, wanting not to be recognized by them, but wanting to see that part of my past is still there. The last time I was in, I stood in the back in an aisle surrounded by tall wooden shelves full of cowboy clothing and enameled metal cookware and I overheard one of the owners up front. He was talking with a woman at the bar about taking a vacation in Ireland and other international trips. It was a far cry from the old bookstore culture of low-paid clerks who went to the local beaches.

I am saying that this coast is full of contradictions for me. It was not always what it is for me now. It never really was an ideal. It used to be unfamiliar. It scared me, belonged to other people, was foggy, windy, and far away, and a challenge. Gradually, I began making it mine through many visits back. On each trip, I came here as if to find out what was true and good in my life. When I was first getting to know the woman I have lived with now for sixteen years, our first daytime date was a trip to the ocean where we had lunch and threw a frisbee. It mattered a great deal to us to find that we each liked the beach. On our ride back, we waited for a long time for gas at a pump beside a coastside restaurant with large blue windows facing toward the sea. That restaurant is gone now, but in my mind I see it clearly, and I see a pink and gray decorated hippie school bus that was parked in front of us for that long half hour while we waited.

My younger brother made this coast his, too. I found out only after his death that his favorite place to go in the whole world was the small flat town of Pescadero. I often imagine him there still, walking around with his camera. He liked to take pictures of nothing happening, of small town Americana, of empty tables set with old silverware and thick round plates in all-night restaurants, of the plain things in life, always in black and white. My brother died eleven years ago; his death was a probable suicide; he was hit by a train. Last winter, to mark the date of his death—he died on a Monday after Thanksgiving—the Tuesday after, I drove down to Pescadero. I wanted to walk through the flat town with its few grid streets and see what my brother once saw and liked, then have lunch at the brown-shingled Pescadero restaurant, sit at the counter, order soup, and think about my brother. I wanted his death not to be in vain.

But I thought I would stop first at the Pescadero Marsh, a wildlife preserve just off the coast highway near the town. I had heard there were wintering birds there. I doubted my brother had been to the marsh, but I wanted to see the birds, and I went because I have found the places where birds live to be reassuring—tranquil, overlooked, out-of-the way natural places, especially the low wetlands. I had never been to the Pescadero Marsh before, and I was anxious about my trip down. Would there be birds? Would the coast be beautiful? Would it be too much changed? Would thinking about my brother upset me? How much of my past would come flooding back to me this time—those old lovers on the beaches, the time I collected sand dollars on the beach before moving to the Southwest. I had thought I would take one as a present to the woman I was going to stay with in Albuquerque while finding a place to live. I never gave it to her, but I did drive cross-country with that sand dollar in the front seat of my car reminding me of where I came from.

It was a foggy morning and an overcast day as I drove down the coast highway to remember my brother. The fog lifted as I neared the marsh. I parked my car in a beach parking lot and walked along the shore. The wind was severe; the ocean was a deep blue with many white-capped waves. I walked on the beach for a long time, then climbed over driftwood, under a bridge, over large rocks, up through ice plant and sand dunes covered with scrubby green vegetation. Then I paused and looked back at the bridge over the inlet to the marsh and remembered when that bridge was a narrow flat wooden bridge rather than the large arching concrete structure I saw now. I remembered a Sunday morning twenty years ago when I came here and the sun was very warm and I felt alone but very good. I had walked the beach until I reached the driftwood, then turned back. I think I felt good because there was a woman I was looking forward to being close with at that time, although it did not work out in the end.

I now climbed to the top of a sand dune and looked inland toward a broad wooded hillside in the distance that seemed to bound the marsh on the inland edge. The marsh that spread out before me seemed just a mass of low-lying reeds, dirt, some trees, patches of still water, and a larger more open pond farther back. I began to walk along a path leading deeper into the marsh toward the hillside. The ocean, the highway, the bridge all receded behind me. The air became quite still, but it was very noisy. The racket was caused, I soon gathered, by thousands of ducks—black, green, brown, yellow— moving about amongst the tall brown and green rushes and the waterways. The ducks took to the air frightened and flew away when I stepped near them. I saw egrets—large white birds with broad flapping wings that make them look like angels as they fly. This marsh was teaming with life. I stood and watched, fascinated.

I had never known there was a marsh here. I had seen a pond to the side of the highway, but for twenty years, I had ignored it and simply walked on the beach from one end to the other and back. I never thought going inland would be worth it. Now I wondered what all the ducks were doing here. I thought there were probably people who could tell the different kinds of ducks from one another. I wished I was one of those people. I wanted more big birds—herons and egrets—and fewer ducks, for the big birds were more dramatic and easier for me to see. But the point was that I was now engaged, debating my past less than which birds I liked. I walked farther into the marsh and was amazed at the extent of it. Half of Pescadero, it seemed to me, was taken up by this marsh. It was set in a broad basin between the sea and the town. It was big enough so that small boats moved around on parts of it farther from me, although near me no boats were allowed, only the reeds and birds.

This was another world—wild, protected, a sanctuary full of clattering ducks, with paths for people overgrown with brush, an occasional bench, signs saying to keep off the regrowing vegetation. Eucalyptus trees seemed to emerge from the bog as I walked. Poison oak was everywhere, along with those tall brown reeds in which were hidden so many kinds of birds. I walked farther in on the path and saw standing near me a great blue heron with a dignified gray body and long legs. I stared at it through my binoculars for some time, and it stared at me. I felt I had found a special place where I could go. I thought my brother had not been here, that he had only been in town, although I did not really know. But this marsh seemed too unruly for him, too noisy. I imagined him where it was quiet. This was my place. I was the only one here. I started to get very warm and suddenly I felt very tired. An hour-and-a-half after I had come, I walked out of the Pescadero Marsh. I climbed over the dunes, under the bridge, and walked back along the beach to my car. Then I drove into the tiny town of Pescadero as I had planned.

I had lunch—soup and bread—in the by now nearly empty restaurant with its pine-panelled walls and its glowing formica counter. Then I took a walk through the flat streets of my brother's town. I did not know exactly where he had gone or what he had liked and I felt frustrated that I could not know. As I walked, I kept looking around, wondering what he had seen. I passed an elementary school. He liked small kids. Maybe he liked that school. I passed small, square wooden houses set back in deep front yards that were planted with a few flowers and spread with children's play things, or odd statuary. The landscape was very flat, the scale low. I passed a blacksmith's shop in a dark, weathered barnlike building. I began feeling that I was invading other people's worlds, and when I kept failing to know what my brother saw, I headed back. The sky was clouding over.

Then on impulse, I turned down a side street where I saw a small old graveyard on a grassy hillside. Thin white tombstones sat gently behind a low wrought-iron fence. I thought my brother must have gone there. He liked things like graveyards. I had always wanted to tell him to go to Colma and Daly City, the graveyard capital of this area where the rolling hills are full of tombs for miles. I thought he'd enjoy walking around there. But I never had told him.

I turned back without going into the delicate Pescadero cemetery or walking around among the plaques. I continued back to the commercial street of town, bought a loaf of sourdough bread in a grocery, a jar of ollalieberry jam in the restaurant, and started home. As I drove out toward the main coast highway, I passed the basin where the Pescadero Marsh lay. I knew it was there but it was hardly distinguishable.

A couple of months later, I took my lover down with me to see the marsh. We parked by the beach, climbed under the bridge and over the dunes and reached the path where the reeds and wetlands stretched out before us, but the marsh was silent. There were no ducks. There was no overwhelming clatter. No birds flew away as soon as I stepped near them. The sky was blue, the feeling peaceful but invigorating. It was a beautiful, but quiet, empty marsh that day. What I had seen a mere two months earlier was no longer there. How easy it is to miss the noise of those quiet places. I tried to explain, to tell my lover what was missing, but really it was missing only for me. No marsh, no tree will ever be what it once was, no lost

44

brother regained. These things are hard to share. Yet that boisterous marsh is there; the coast around Half Moon Bay stretches long and uninterrupted by the sea; my brother, who liked all-night restaurants and who lured me down to Pescadero to take a look around again, is still very present in my mind.

PART 2

Inner Visions

FIVE

Lesbian Invisibility

Reflecting on disappearing geographic landscapes soon led me to think about disappearing lesbian landscapes. This story about looking for lesbians at a folk music festival highlights for me the evanescence of lesbian realities: they are sometimes visible but then are quickly gone. What would happen, I wondered, if lesbianism as a reality were not so fleeting? This story seeks to make visible the contours of an often hidden social landscape.

OF ALL LESBIAN TOPICS, the key to the rest, it seems to me, is that of lesbian invisibility. This is a subject I take so for granted that even to think about it seems a huge undertaking. I am a lesbian. So much hinges on that statement, or on the need to begin with it. Why is it so necessary to say, "I am a lesbian"? Why is it so hard to say? Both the necessity and the difficulty suggest to me the importance of invisibility in lesbian life.

Here are two facts of my own life. The first is that I am always looking for other lesbians—and I am always unsure of whether I am seeing them. They are always disappearing on me, or they appear,

49

but I am not sure for how long they will stay. Is a woman I am seeing now a lesbian for a moment, a year, a few years? Is she a lesbian in private but not in public? Is she a lesbian for life, as I am?

The second fact is that I am always wondering whether I am seen as a lesbian—whether I am visible and what my visibility is taken to mean by others. I wonder not only about what straight people see, but also about what other lesbians see. Do they recognize me as a lesbian, and if so, what kind of a lesbian, and is a lesbian even something one can be anymore? Does the category of lesbianism still exist, or has it disappeared into a postmodern amorphousness of identity, a nonspecific sense of having multiple identities, a "don't pin me down" attitude that adds to a prior strong pull to avoid the stigma of lesbianism, to avoid the persecution that has long caused lesbians to be in the closet? The stigma associated with lesbianism has caused us to blend in, to adopt a protective camouflage—a distinctly female camouflage—as we pass as conventional women, and sometimes as men—all to avoid passing as lesbian. Even with today's more accepting attitudes toward lesbianism, I often feel that these attitudes are only skin deep; they accept the appearance of being a lesbian but not the underlying reality.

I want to discuss that reality and some of the struggles with invisibility that I have experienced and noticed. Why do others disappear? Why do I do so myself? Here is a story about lesbian invisibility—a set of images I have found helpful for thinking about why lesbianism is so often something no longer there, an invisibility in the social landscape.

A few weeks ago, I went to an outdoor summer folk music festival on the Pacific coast of Canada. It was held in a scenic park next to a bay, on an expanse of grassy fields and rolling hillsides. The view across the water was of mountains—brown in the near distance, snow-capped peaks farther back. The park had open lawns and tree-shaded areas, and ponds with tall rushes and ducks floating on them. Spaced out over the hillsides or under the trees were half a dozen small stages, each covered with a red and white striped tent top to protect performers from rain or sun. During the day, people would go to these different performance areas to listen to music (3,000 to 6,000 attended the festival on each of three days). In the evenings, we gathered on blankets in a central meadow and listened to a four-hour-long concert in which many acts performed on a broad front stage under a colorful arching frame. As the sun went down, the stage became lit with red, blue, and purple lights. The sunlight lasted until almost 10 P.M.; the crowd dispersed by 11, led quietly to exits by people carrying candle-lit lanterns in the dark.

The days were full of people walking around and sitting on the grass listening to music—gospel, traditional, old left, women's music, rebel voices, bluegrass, folk music from many countries. This was my first visit to the festival. I liked seeing the many blankets laid out in front of the central evening stage. Each day people got to the festival grounds early in the morning when the gates opened to place their blankets on the grass end-to-end as close to the stage as possible, marking a place to come back to for the evening concert. By late morning, the sea of blankets stretched far back on the field. By evening, especially Saturday evening, the blankets stretched nearly to the shore along the bay. Looking at this sea of blankets, I saw plastic tarps, often blue, lying exposed or beneath the blankets, and then the expanse of squares of so many colors. Many of them were brightly patterned Mexican blankets with brown, blue, and red stripes and diamond-shaped designs. There were sleeping bags unrolled and laid out, plaid-flannel side up; blankets from kids' beds at home; western-style blankets with bold black stripes; floral home-sweet-home style blankets; solid colors; old faded bedspreads.

The large expanse in front of the stage, made up of all these blanket squares, looked like a quilt. It was like the AIDS quilt, I thought, but without the deliberately embroidered panels, without the specific names of people, usually men, who had died of AIDS. No, this quilt, like the experience I had during those two-and-a-half days, was a different kind—unnamed, invisible, an anonymous quilt that was not formally announced or designed—a women's quilt. For this festival was attended, I was to find, in large part by women, and to an unusual degree by lesbians. It was not a "women's music" festival, nor was it a lesbian music festival, but women were its largest visible subgroup, making up at least two-thirds of the total; and of these, a significant number were lesbians, accounting for perhaps 25 percent of the women, perhaps for nine hundred people on Saturday when the biggest crowds came. Or so it seemed to me. I must add that qualifier. For there is always the question of whether I am seeing lesbians when they are not there.

Is a woman I am seeing who looks to me like a lesbian really one?, I wonder. Is she a lesbian if she does not call herself a lesbian? What if she does not tell me about it? What are the criteria? How do we know? At the festival, I just took the risk; I relied on what I saw. I imagined lesbians into the scene and that is the important point. There is also a point about respect for such imagining and for the type of world it creates. By seeing lesbians, I created a lesbian world in my mind, a world of my own people, a world built out of my needs. It was a challenge, however, for the lesbians at this folk music festival were not highly visible. They were often there one moment and gone the next, leaving me wondering about whether in fact I had seen them.

For these were not in-your-face, swaggering, hair standing-on-end lesbians, not lesbians in overalls, or even blue jeans—the weather called for shorts—not baseball cap lesbians. They were not lesbians who looked like men or smoked pipes or cigars, or wore ties or tuxedos or men's trousers, or who hung on each others' shoulders and roamed bare-breasted through the grassy hillsides. They did not sit in front of the performance tents holding hands or smooching and saying "right on" or calling for their favorite performers to sing lesbian songs. Nor did they loudly cheer whenever a potential lesbian innuendo was made from a stage.

Quite the contrary, these were quiet lesbians. They were dressed for the most part in neat, khaki shorts and tee shirts and small, front-brimmed hats. Although they had short hair, they sat a nice distance apart and when they were in groups, they did not talk loudly to one another. They did not give each other big lesbian bear hugs or engage in group gropes; they blended in. The straight women tended to stand out, with their hippy clothing, their flowing, filmy skirts, their unkempt long, loose hair; while the lesbians were more tailored in dress, as if they felt less freedom to be expressive and needed to keep things more under control. They looked a bit like Dinah Shore lesbians—women's golf circuit lesbians—but without the gold jewelry and makeup and probably they were quieter. Maybe, to most of the world, they would not even look like lesbians, but I was on the watch. I had been told they were here, that for quite a few years, this folk music festival was a place to go for lesbians—mostly from Canada and the United States, but also from other countries.

I walked around the festival grounds looking carefully for signs. How close did a woman sit to the woman next to her? How direct was the feeling in the air between them? Lesbians, it seemed to me, had a directness. There was not a layer of puff between them that kept them apart. I looked for a few inches of greater than usual closeness in the way two women sat next to each other on a blanket. I looked for a quietness between them, a seriousness in how they regarded each other. I watched for brief expressions of intimacy followed by a holding back. I looked at women's clothes—how they were worn and how the women moved. I looked for an absence of effeminacy, and for whether a woman had an upright bodily stance. I looked for women holding hands or dancing close together. I looked for intimate embraces, but I did not see any. My lover and I held hands a lot, and occasionally we kissed, but I felt we were in a minority. I felt, in general, a lesbian presence at the festival but also a lesbian invisibility.

I thought about how Canadian politeness might account for the invisibility, but that there were probably other sources as well. Twice I saw straight women breastfeeding their babies in public, carefully taking out a breast from a soft blouse and then putting it back. The lesbians did not breastfeed, or did not bring babies, or those with tiny infants did not come.

I saw, of course, only a small slice of what was there. Yet the straight women seemed to me to talk more; they were more chatty, more effusive, although within limits; they filled up the space more. The lesbians were watchful, probably like I was, because this was not our home turf. It was clearly a straight people's festival with some lesbians in it. There was no way to count exactly how many. At one particular concert on women's work, I felt I was seeing many lesbians— sitting on the grass, greeting each other with brief hugs and short kisses, the sleeves of their tee shirts neatly rolled up, muscle style, several earrings in an ear, serious sunglasses, tank top shirts, a thin leather armband here and there, a carefully drawn tattoo on a tanned shoulder. A woman in front of me had on a tee shirt with the sleeves rolled up, dark glasses, short brown hair. With a cock of her head— her head was held straight—she seemed to be saying, "I am a lesbian and I am sitting next to another woman who is a lesbian—maybe she's my friend, or my lover or former lover, and the woman sitting next to her is a friend of hers, or maybe her former lover, or her former lover's ex's lover." There seemed to be an unstated, "We're lesbians, but you would not necessarily know it. We're discreet."

Some of the lesbians had on shirts that said "Staff" on the back, so I assumed they had authority and they seemed imposing to me. I always find lesbians I do not know who dress or act tough or cool or mannish to be intimidating. Then an individual will speak and I will find her friendly, and I will consider that there is probably a reason for the intimidating appearance. It's a sign, an announcement, "Keep Out." I make such signs myself, announcing by how I walk and move and dress that I am a lesbian and that this means keep your hands off. I do want some hands on me, but not in public, and in spite of the toughness or aloofness I may convey. I think lesbians know that no one is aloof, that there is always a way to reach or touch another woman, that the toughest-looking lesbian is often the softest, that it's the sharp, straight, femme woman who is to be feared. She is willing to be touched by a man but not a woman. She's really tough; she's closed off. I wouldn't want to be her, I feel. I wonder, how can she survive? Isn't it a life of deprivation?

But in public I don't say this, and the lesbians at the Canadian folk music festival did not say it. They sat patiently and listened to the many concerts and sometimes they danced, usually individually, in the aisles, and although they clapped loudly for certain acts, they kept a lot inside. They did not disturb the surface of events, or challenge the way the scene was set. The few men present often had graying beards and looked like survivors from the old and new left.

At one point, I was sitting in front of a stage with its red and white striped tent top. The sun was warm, and to my delight, a group of young Australian dykes appeared. They jumped up before the microphones full of raw energy. No one said the word dyke or lesbian, but it seemed apparent; they had short, spiky hair and one had blue hair. They stood before everyone and generally cut up, had a good time, sang about women loving women, and had a key song with the line, "I will kneel right down and bow my head and let you let me in." How truly lesbian, I felt, relieved, happy for the use of the words; this was not male sex, nor a woman's version of male sex. They sang their songs with great joy and abandon and had a trumpet and soprano sax player who belted things out, and electric guitars, and they were real loud, not genteel folksingers, not respectful of the milieu.

As I listened to this group, I found myself smiling and laughing in the sun in that large crowd of several hundred women—only some of them lesbians, but quite a few, quiet lesbians, applauding loudly, sometimes getting up to dance on the grassy hillside. The band got louder and a gray-haired, gray-bearded man in front of me got up and walked away. A man and woman farther up front near the stage soon got up and left quickly together. We were thinning them out. I thought it made sense. This was not their music, but I also thought they missed the best part.

The Australian dyke group was exceptional for me because in the other concerts, no one had sung decidedly lesbian songs. I had heard that in prior years, there were lesbian performers who did use the "L" word, and if there were enough of them any year, there was a more palpable lesbian presence. Once they had a performance workshop called "The 'L' Word," but not this year. This year, I heard the word from a stage at only one event in three days, when a woman who played with a man and called herself "Difficult Women" performed. But it seemed to me she was probably bisexual, not lesbian. I heard that a straight, male left-wing folksong writer had sung a lesbian song in his set, using the "L" word, but that was all. There were lesbian performers who remained unidentified.

One morning, an African American women's group sang gospel and traditional African music so joyful that a large number of people swayed and danced in the sun and under the trees while listening. Who was a lesbian among these dancers? I thought as I watched the women around me. One, in particular, had on brown hiking boots, cut-off tan tight-fitting shorts, and a white tank-top shirt. She had a thick black belt on her shorts, and long, wavy blond hair. Don't be fooled by the hair, I thought, watch how she moves. Look at that belt—it's too wide; it's too black for a straight woman's belt. She's too tanned, too present. But really it is hard to tell. Just because I want to be surrounded by lesbians and because I often think I see them does not mean they are there.

One day at lunchtime, I went to a food stand and bought a veggie Sloppy Joe—a big pile of reddish brown hamburger-looking food that was scooped onto a long hot dog bun. I brought it over to a shady area to eat it in comfort while listening to a concert with my lover. She had also brought a sandwich. We found a spot beneath a tree. As we started to sit down, two women sitting directly in front of us turned around and smiled. "Big sandwich—that looks good," one of them said to me. "Where did you get it?" "At the vegetarian stand near the side gate," I told her. I looked up from my sandwich into the face of a woman who wore wire-rimmed aviator glasses and had short, graying brown hair and a soft body. She sat next to a woman who was older than she, whose hair was more white but also short, and who had a similar full-bodied butch appearance. They have to be lesbians, I thought. Who else would be interested in my sandwich? Who else would turn around and smile so broadly—upon seeing my lover and me, both, too, with short hair, both butch, both very serious about our lunch, and about each other. A third woman was with these two, but I did not feel she was a lesbian, although you never really know. I thought the women were probably Canadian. They soon turned back around to listen to the concert.

As I sat listening and eating my lunch, I looked at the backs of their heads very closely. I watched as the two I thought were lesbians turned to each other to share a few words. I invented lives for them. I imagined that one of them was a librarian, and the other a school teacher, or maybe in construction. Maybe their straight friend was also a librarian; maybe she was a lesbian. Maybe the older lesbian was retired. She had very strong glasses and very white hair. I so much wanted them to turn around again and talk to me, but they never did. Eventually I got up and left and I felt a loss. For a brief moment, I had felt a sense of lesbian presence, and then it was gone.

On Saturday, the weather was very hot. By afternoon, the sun was beating down, the air was still and muggy and people were sweating. To cool off, my lover and I went to get water from a spigot that protruded from the ground near a pond. Seven or eight people were waiting in line there to fill their plastic water bottles, or to pour the water from the bottles over their heads and their bodies to cool themselves down. Occasionally someone just stuck their head under the faucet. When I got in line, I saw, standing in front of me, a woman in cut-off blue-jean shorts that were held up with a broad, black leather belt. She wore a thick, black leather armband with many steel studs in it, and leather combat-style boots, and she was bare-breasted. She was certainly a lesbian, I thought. Who else would expose her breasts in this way? The straight women at the festival demurely took out a breast while feeding a baby, and then tucked it back in—a sign of nurturant femaleness, not of lesbianism.

I was so glad to see this bare-breasted woman. I felt suddenly happy and free, as I had while listening to the Australian dyke group perform with their loud trumpet player and their spiky hair. I looked at the woman's breasts, trying to seem like I was not looking. I investigated every inch of her. She was daring to do what others would not do. It was legal here in Canada for women to bare their breasts in public. I knew it was what lesbians did at women's gatherings like the Michigan Womyn's Music Festival. But I had seen no other bare-breasted women here. The breasts of the woman in the cut-off blue jeans looked a lot like mine, I thought; they were about the same size. She definitely did not need a bra, or even a shirt. The day was very hot. I thought about how brave she was, because other people would look at her and stare, as I had. She had to be able to ignore them. She had to have a purpose and stay focused on her own life.

I wanted to go up to her, to say thank you. I wanted to say, "How great you are!" I wanted to give her a high sign, a quiet, semi-private acknowledgment between us, a wave of my hand. But that would be calling attention. That would be singling her out, not letting her bare breasts go by as if unnoticed, as if, of course, this were natural, as if everybody did it. It would make her feel more uncomfortable. It would suggest I was staring, that I was watching her and appreciating her breasts along with her black belt and that studded dog collar on her arm.

I said nothing. I watched her bend over to fill her large, plastic water bottle. Did she know how I felt? I wondered. I hoped she knew. How could she not know? One look at me and she'd know.

And then she gave me a chance. She had seemed to me nervous while filling her bottle, and then she dropped it. It fell from her hands, mostly full, onto the muddy, grassy ground beneath the spigot and rolled downhill toward me. I quickly bent down, grabbed it, and handed it back up to her. Now the bottle was muddy from the ground. I hoped she would wash it off. She accepted it back with a thank you, as if she were truly grateful, beyond the bottle, I hoped. I hoped she would know what I had meant by so quickly returning it to her. I knew all along that she could pick up her own water bottle. I hoped she knew by my picking it up and handing it to her that I, too, was a lesbian, and that I thought she was, and that I was so very grateful to her for going around bare-breasted.

I like to look at women's breasts, many women's breasts. I would like to go without a shirt myself, but it makes me self-conscious. I like especially to look at lesbians' breasts—for the sense of freedom implied and the sense that these breasts are not entirely off limits to me, as straight women's breasts often seem to be.

I could see that the woman with the armband was still nervous. I felt I was such a coward. She half-washed off the mud from her water bottle, filled it the remaining way, capped it, and walked off away from me into the crowd. Later that day, I saw her again. I was sitting on a bench under some trees. She was walking on a path nearby with several friends. I saw her bare breasts and again felt glad. I wanted to run over and thank her, but I stayed where I was.

Lesbian invisibility, the theme repeats. That quiet, suppressed, polite, fading-into-the-background lesbian presence at the Canadian folk music festival was not unusual. But what an image it was for me—the looming brown mountains, the bright blue sky, the bay, the lesbians. What are they afraid of? I wondered and asked my lover many times. Why does this happen? What if we danced close and sat closer and yelled out requests for lesbian songs? What if we dropped the word lesbian into every other sentence? What if we stopped disappearing? What if being only women was enough?

Why didn't the lesbians at the festival assert themselves more as lesbians? Why didn't I? What is the fear? I thought at the time it was that the straight people would leave. The men would go and the women would follow and then there would no longer be this folk festival. There would remain only lesbians to make our own festival—smaller, poorer, with more visible lesbians in it, full of the conflicts, the joys, the breasts of lesbian communities. There are such festivals and I have been to some of them, but that is not quite my point. Then there would no longer be this festival. There would have to be a new world—one where lesbianism did not just fit in but defined things, determined how we related. What if lesbians no longer blended in, invisibly supporting the straight world, but defined a different way? What if others blended into a lesbian world, or simply saw it and learned from it, if it changed them. It was hard, but exciting, for me to imagine.

I had one other experience at the Canadian folk festival that bears telling, I think, because of the connections it points to between worlds. On the last day, I went to a concert called "The Solidarity Workshop." It featured two straight women who sang harmonies together a cappella, one soulful African American woman, one sensitive left-wing man, and two old-time leftist men—one of them out of the British labor tradition and the other out of the American West, a storyteller with a long, white beard and a long, white pony tail down his back. The two older men had deep, big voices and tended to dominate. The African American woman was thrilling and independent. Many people filled out the crowd that day, making for a very large audience in the same performance area where the afternoon before, the Australian dyke group had played. Now the crowd had more older people in it—more men with beards and balding heads and women with flowing skirts who sat with them. The lesbians present seemed scattered here and there. The crowd felt very dense to me. The solidarity theme—drawing from the old union movement—felt overwhelming, backed by the powerful voices of the old men and by, I felt, a bit of guilt. The concert ran well over the time alotted for it, and this festival was one in which events ran strictly on time.

Toward the end, there were two finale songs, "Rolling Home Together" and "Solidarity Forever." The two older men, along with the others on the stage, led the large, very involved audience in singing them. The crowd joined in increasingly and sang with much feeling. At one point in "Rolling Home Together," led specifically by the British man with the deep voice and years of labor movement experience, there was a line where I heard he used the word "their"—as a sub-stitute, I felt, for what had once been "his." That word stood out to me, perhaps because these men reminded me of my father. He had cared very much about the union movement. The ideology of labor—of people being of value and rising up against capitalism and the bosses—was a central part of my upbringing. I suddenly thought my father might have done something like that, changed the word to put the women in. I looked at my lover, standing by my side, whom I have been with for seventeen years, and I wished my father had been able to meet her. I felt sure he would have liked her, and I missed him then, and I wanted to bring him back to life. Suddenly, I was crying deeply heavy sobs that made me feel out of balance, like I ought to sit down. But most of my crying was internal.

Then "Solidarity Forever" started and soon the whole large crowd of hundreds was standing and singing as if they had been asked to. I saw that my lover turned to an old man standing next to her, a slim, slightly bent-over man with a scruffy white beard—maybe he was in his late seventies—and she reached out her hand to him. At first, he shrugged it off—he didn't need her hand—and then he took it. See-ing her, I turned to a woman on my left, a straight woman in a billowy skirt and peach-colored blouse. I reached out my hand and she took it gladly. We sang and swayed and cried and soon a woman who had been sitting in front of me came quickly and got between me and the woman in the peach-colored blouse. She held out her hands to both of us, making the circle, or the extension of the arms, wider. And then everyone was singing and beaming and crying, and I was sobbing and beaming and crying and I wished I wasn't. I wished my sister was there. I wished that all that old left stuff didn't make me so uncom-fortable. I wished that I could truly feel the solidarity they all seemed to feel. But I could not. I was too aware of feeling like a lesbian and a woman and like these were men and it was a man's tradition and I missed my father very much. I knew I was indebted to him, but somehow it wasn't as simple as it appeared to be. Nor is lesbian soli-darity simple for me, but it is something I have come to on my own.

Later, I briefly talked to the woman to my left, whose hand I had first reached for, and my lover told me that as the crowd split up, she heard a man in back of her say to someone near him, "I wish my daddy were here." I wondered, would it be the same thing for his daddy to be here as it would be for mine? Would it surprise our fathers if they came here and they were among lesbians—standing linking the generations, reaching out to the people on the sides of them? But lesbians are so invisible, would they even know we were here? I was told later that lesbians made up a large part of the volunteer staff at the festival, but I did not notice that at the time; it was not easy to see them.

The next day, we were finally on our way home, two women with luggage checking through Customs and sitting in a Canadian airport waiting for our flight. In the bar where we sat having a snack, the people at the other tables were quiet, except for two loud American men in Stetson cowboy hats who yelled to each other across their tables about business in Arizona. I wanted not to be an American just then, but I did want to be a lesbian. I knew I was not the same as these men, but it was harder for me to know who I was.

An image suddenly came to mind. I remembered that quilt laid out in the very center of the grassy festival grounds made up of those many brightly colored, patterned blankets, that quilt with no name and no organizer, but with a purpose. I had liked the way it just sat there. People didn't even know to appreciate it; they stepped all over it. But I saw it, briefly, laid down each morning, taken up each night. That is how I felt about the lesbians, that I saw them briefly, as I see my own lesbian self briefly. Occasional lesbian exposures seem all I can manage, yet I always want there to be more, and more than just the surface signs—the clothes, the style of a woman's hair, the suggestion that an armband or a belt stands for a lesbian life. I want more expression of what is beneath the surface–of the feelings inside, the statements that are never quite made. I want to know, What are the inner realities we so hide and protect by making them invisible?

Like that beautiful quilt made up of blankets laid out on the festival grass, we are stepped on because people don't see, and even if they saw us, there would still be needs for protection. What are these needs? Why the invisibility? Is it necessary? Will it always be this way? What underlying fears cause the disappearances?

Lesbianism, for me, is like a soft center, a world unto itself that would not in fact survive total integration with straight society. It is a world made up of needs women have of one another, that I have of other women. It is real and, at the same time, an ideal of comfort, retreat, female independence, female love. Lesbian invisibility is, I think, a statement of the need to protect a lesbian world, of the need for a lesbian separation—the need to draw a boundary around ourselves in order to build something different.

My lesbianism is a very private desire. I find it hard to make that private experience into something public, to lay it out before people who will not identify with it enough to understand it. So I, like other women, often withdraw.

Much as I was bothered by all the lesbian disappearances at the folk festival, I know well that there are reasons for the disappearances. I know, too, that I prize the special secret world of indirect lesbian signs, symbols, and assumed meanings. I prize the sense of having a shadow reality that I see but others do not. I like the feeling of creating a world anew. Yet I worry about that world disappearing—not that we won't tell everyone else we are lesbians, but that we won't create the spaces needed to tell each other, and then we won't know who we are. I will feel then that all the secrets I have will just have to stay within me. So I write. I try to pin it down, I try to create through my imagination a lesbian world behind what is normally seen. My sense is that I am not alone in doing this, that lesbians actively imagine and invent other lesbians all the time, constantly looking for signs—a black studded armband, or short hair, a private smile, a certain attentiveness. Thus out of the blue on a grassy field, a lost lesbian landscape may appear.

SIX

I See Her in My Mind

The time spent in an intimate relationship may be momentary, but especially if it is a lesbian relationship, the impact may linger long after the intimacy is gone. In this story I recall a relationship from my past that I often return to in my mind, seeking a deeply felt comfort and a sense of home.

LAST FALL, I WAS TRAVELING in the Southwest with my lover when we stopped for dinner one night at a roadside Mexican restaurant. It had black wrought-iron bars on the windows and multicolored Christmas lights still strung on the eaves from the year before. As we stepped inside, the restaurant looked cavernous, dim, and empty. Then through a broad archway, I saw the main dining room, lit brightly with a soft yellowish light. In the rear of this room, at the only occupied table, sat a woman whose shoulderlength white-gray hair glowed and shook like tinsel. She was speaking to a smaller dark-haired woman sitting across from her, whose back was to me. Her eyes gleamed. I lost my breath for a moment.

I instinctively stepped back after my first glance in the direction of these two women and hid behind a wooden post to the side of the entry arch. Standing there in the half-dark, I wondered if the woman with the glowing hair was indeed Bess, a woman important to me years ago, or just someone who looked like her. Bess's hair used to be honey-colored, but this woman looked so familiar. The sideways tilt of her head was characteristic. I thought that my quick stepping backward meant it was indeed Bess, and that the woman across from her was her lover of many years, Marie. When I am not sure if a person I am seeing is someone I know, I move closer for a further look. Yet I had withdrawn and was standing as if frozen. My lover, Hannah, had walked over and was now standing beside me looking at a menu.

"See anything here you could eat?" she asked, her tone at once practical yet expressing concern for me, a tone so like Hannah, who is alert and caring.

It had been eight years since I last saw Bess, at another restaurant and another table. Hannah was with me then too, and Marie was with Bess, and it was an awkward dinner. I have never understood why the break between Bess and me occurred. I do not understand how the past between myself and another woman can suddenly be gone.

I lived in New Mexico fourteen years ago, not here but in a town several hours south. At that time, Bess provided a second home for me. She was my comfort, my stability. I was teaching at the state university for a year, and when my job ended, I began moving from place to place, unsure of where I would be living next. Bess offered me her house as my mailing address during my moves. She gave me a key so I could check my mail and so I would have a place to go when I needed to run away. When the male lover of a woman I was soon living with came to visit, when the nights were hard, I would get in my car and drive to Bess's house, even if I did not go in. I needed a destination, another home, a different kind of reality.

Bess's house, where she lived with Marie, was a small adobe in the old part of town. The house was square, low-lying, earthen-colored and hidden behind a thick adobe wall. It seemed to disappear into the flat dusty landscape all around it, where other houses hidden behind other walls lay close to the earth on narrow streets. The house had a bare yard in back where Bess and Marie kept their four dogs. Inside, the space was largely one room—a big, comfortable living room with a log-beamed ceiling, its walls lined with books, its wooden floor spread with worn, woven Indian-style rugs. Pueblo pots were placed around on high shelves. A boarded-up fireplace in the back of the living room did not work, but a rounded white kiva fireplace in the kitchen did, and after being used it left a soft piñon fir smell that pervaded the entire house.

Often I visited Bess and Marie in the evenings and we would sit talking in the living room, the dogs and their two cats wandering in and out. We sat in the one half of that room that had light, Bess on a square comfortable chair, bookshelves climbing the wall behind her, a standing reading lamp throwing light from behind on her honey-blond hair which, even then graying, was pulled back and tied low behind her head. Marie and I sat across from her on a small couch. We each talked personally, though with some distance. My main relationship was with Bess, although of necessity, it involved Marie, who accepted the intimacy of our relationship and I often wondered why. I liked Marie. She was down to earth and, like Bess, generous.

As we talked, both Bess and Marie often gave me advice. They were somewhat older than me. Sometimes I had dinner with them at large American-style restaurants, where they often ate. On weekends, they showed me around the local area and took me with them to crafts fairs and out-of-the-way desert towns, the three of us riding high up in the cab of Bess's white Ford pickup. I felt accepted by them.

On weekdays, I often stopped by Bess's house to check my mail when no one was home. I would look in on the dogs, sit in the coolness of the darkened living room, watch television, and rest.

Sometimes I took care of the animals when Bess and Marie went away. When the three of us were together in the evenings, we often talked about people we knew, especially other lesbians, and women who became involved with lesbians. One of these was a straight woman I was becoming close with who had touched deep feelings in me and promised to help me make my life better. My relationship with her was important for me, emotionally difficult, and mostly kept secret. Bess encouraged me in this relationship and helped me to deal with my emotions concerning it, which was something I very much needed. I often felt that Bess was sharing the relationship, invisibly becoming involved with the straight woman too, though perhaps it was a more general sharing of an intimacy, as lesbians often do.

My straight friend, Anna, was quite different from Bess. She was more volatile in personality, more dramatic, a fantasy mother to me, a woman I was constantly questing after. Bess was understated, more suppressed, responsive to me in a low-key way. I would spend time with Anna, then go to Bess for support. I think that my image of Bess has come to stand for my feelings about both of these women. It has come to stand for that time in my life—a restless, lonely, adventuresome time that I often feel I should be living in again. I feel I should be the same "free spirit," the same undetermined, wandering type of woman—available, visiting, new in the area, living on the edge of others' lives, a woman whom others seemed interested in.

My relationship with Bess began rather slowly with a chance meeting. I first became friendly with her one weekend during my first spring in town when we were helping a lesbian couple we both knew move. A group of women were carrying lamps and tables out to a large truck when I arrived. Bess looked up and seemed glad to see me. That night, I visited her at her house and met Marie, who seemed welcoming. A few weeks later, when I went on a camping trip, Bess and Marie came by to feed a stray calico cat who had been hanging around the house where I was living near the university. That summer, I housesat out near the mountain behind town. Bess came and slept there several nights when I was away so that the calico cat, now adopted by me and about to have kittens, would not give birth alone. I was moved by her willingness to do that. Bess encouraged me to keep my cat, who waited to have her kittens until late the night I got back.

When a few weeks afterward, I moved in with Anna, taking with me my cat and her four kittens in a large cardboard box, Bess was very much with me in the back of my mind. The house where I now began to live with Anna was a modern mock-adobe out on the sandy mesa north of town. I remember calling Bess one night from Anna's kitchen to tell her I had seen a puppy at the pound, but I was uncertain about whether to get him. He was a small black male and I had gone in search of a medium-sized female dog. "Go get him," Bess said to me bluntly, her voice seeming to emerge from out of nowhere on the other end of the phone. "Be there first thing in the morning before they open or they may kill your dog." How did she know, I wondered. I felt she had recognized in my voice that this small black dog I could not decide about was one I already felt was mine.

I often felt Bess knew what I most wanted. After I had been living with Anna for a few months, I was debating whether to move to California, since there were no academic positions for me in New Mexico. I met Bess one afternoon at a McDonald's to ask her advice. Sitting across a small table from me, a window behind her, she looked at me seriously. "I think you should stay here," she said. "You've begun something important with Anna. You should give yourself a chance to find out where it leads." This was what I had most wanted to hear, but I could not say it to myself. Did Bess want me to stay for her too? I wondered.

I soon began writing stories, and I showed some of my initial writing to Bess. She liked my writing. One day when we were out for lunch at a local park, I asked her about a story I had just revised. "I liked the first version better," she said. "It sounds more like how you speak." I was glad for this affirmation of myself. That day as we sat on the grass and talked—about my writing, about personal odds and ends—I looked into Bess's eyes and I felt we were the only two people in the world, and I felt that Bess cared about me.

She and I often sought out such small moments of being alone. One evening, I met her at her house and we walked over to the Old Town commercial area and wandered the streets in the dark, looking into the lighted windows of closed stores where silver jewelry and pottery glistened in the displays. Bess pointed out to me small carved turquoise figures of animals that she liked. We walked close together for some time on the narrow alleys and talked about our lives. Before leaving, we stood for a long time under a street lamp, the light shining down softly on us. Bess touched my arm, then she hesitated, and I wanted us not to go back.

Whether I met her at home or out, Bess usually seemed glad to see me, although often she was preoccupied. She was a strange woman. Serious, she held herself at a distance. At the same time, she reached out to me, beckoning me near. Bess was gentle, but she did not have many of the social graces others did. She left uncomfortable silences, said things bluntly. I was drawn to her as if her awkwardness was itself charming.

Once when Anna went back East over Thanksgiving, Bess came out with Marie to visit me so I would not feel lonely. I have photographs of the two of them sitting on the white bench seat next to the fireplace in Anna's living room, looking like two ordinary women— open-faced, friendly, smiling. Bess's eyes glint with her smile, although, as always, I felt she was anxious. That day had a special feel for me. I was suddenly among lesbians in a house where I often felt I ought to be straight. It had snowed outside, which was unusual, the snow dusting the sand, cactus, and pointed yucca with white. I took pictures of that too, and although I can't find them, they stay in my mind.

At Christmastime, Bess invited me to bring Anna along to a small gathering at her house. It was the only time I went somewhere with Anna where people knew of the lesbian nature of our relationship and invited us as a couple because of it. I have photographs of Anna and

me sitting together in Bess and Marie's comfortable living room—
Anna, with a wine glass in her hand, is looking at me affectionately.
Behind us is the boarded up fireplace and, in front of it, a Christmas
tree strung with colored lights and silver tinsel. When I went into
the kitchen that night to refill our drinks, Bess smiled at me. I went
back out to be with Anna, who also smiled. The whole atmosphere
felt cordial. That evening, I felt as if Anna, too, was a lesbian.

Not long afterward, Bess came out to visit me one evening at
Anna's house. We sat talking on the floor of my room on the tan car-
pet. My puppy lay in a small heap of blackness beside us. After a
while, I put my head in Bess's lap and asked her to hold me. She held
me briefly, but she seemed uncomfortable and soon got up and left.
I felt sad. I had expected her to stay longer. I thought maybe she did
not like being in the same house with Anna there. Or perhaps it was
something about me that made her leave.

At one point, Marie had to go back to Kansas to the small town
where her family lived. She flew there and Bess and I drove out a few
days later in Bess's white Ford pickup to bring Marie home and carry
back some family furniture. On the drive, I sat next to Bess in the
cab of her truck. I did not know what to do with the closeness
between us. I reached my arm over toward Bess but then did not
know whether to leave it on her shoulder. She seemed not to know
either. Then she seemed not to want me to go further.

As we drove through the plains of Texas and Oklahoma, the air
felt warm. I remember we stopped for a couple of hours in the very
early morning at a motel near the southern border of Kansas for Bess
to take a shower. I can still see the dawn light coming up behind a
large neon blue sign that said "Motel." I see Bess coming out from the
motel after her shower, the rosy dawn in the hazy blue sky behind her.
She walks up to the truck where I am sitting inside, climbs up into
the cab, and we drive off. In my mind, it's as if that moment stands
for a more general haziness in the sexual relationship between us.

The next night, which we spent in Kansas, Bess stayed with
Marie in a front room of Marie's mother's house. I slept in a room

over the garage out in back. It was a restless night for me. I ached to be with Bess. The next morning, the three of us drove off. I sat on the outside of the bench seat in the truck and felt far away from Bess. Marie sat in the middle between us. We kept stopping and getting out of the truck to make sure the furniture did not blow away in back. The ride home seemed to me to take much longer than the ride there.

Related to that trip in my mind was a time when Bess left her normal life back at home for a few days and stayed in a motel on the southeast edge of town where the road stretches out into the desert. She called me to come visit her there and I stayed with her for a while in that grayish motel room with the two double beds. Bess lay in one of the beds under the covers. I sat in a chair beside her and we talked. A sense of expectancy lay between us. Bess took my hand and held it. I felt she was depressed, or that she wanted to get away from home, or from Marie; she was thinking things over. She had a package of devil's food cakes with her that she ate when she got into the bed, slowly peeling back the cellophane wrapper. To this day, I feel like I would like to eat some. When I left the motel late that afternoon, I stepped into the bright sunlight and looked down from the upper deck at the asphalt parking lot below and the world felt too bright and harsh to me. I wished I were back inside with Bess.

Soon after that, Bess visited me one afternoon where I was house-sitting and we tried to have a regular sexual experience. But it was disappointing. When Bess first arrived, I was standing in the kitchen next to the refrigerator. Then somehow I had taken off my clothes and was lying on the couch in the family room, asking Bess to come be with me. It felt awkward, so we moved into the master bedroom, where I pulled down the shades. I lay next to Bess in the darkness and touched her. She seemed to enjoy it, but she soon turned inward and seemed sad. Afterward, I wished I had not lured us into bed.

Most of the sexuality between us was not in bed, however, but just in the air. When I would stop by at Bess's house in the evenings, I would feel a physical-sexual excitement between myself and Bess, a subdued, understated flirtation. I felt it in the way she looked at me when I arrived, as I stepped into the living room, closing the screen door behind me, closing out the world. Bess smiled at me and was welcoming. I felt the excitement when we passed close to each other briefly touching in the kitchen, or in a knowing glance from Bess from across the living room while we were talking with Marie. I felt it when we stood near each other when we were out, or when we sat across a table at dinner and Bess looked at me. These moments were full of promise for me. They made me shiver, made goose bumps rise up on my back, made my ears get warm, and produced between my legs a soft gently touched feeling, as if an invisible quiver owned me. A nervous softness surrounded me and Bess. The sexuality of our relationship made me feel that Bess cared about me and that there were not barriers between us.

I felt that Bess viewed me with affection, but it was not a simple affection. I think she wanted our relationship to be safe, to be exciting and flattering, but at the same time, undisturbing of other things in each of our lives. She wanted to be helpful to me. And she was. So many times, I went to her to talk about my relationship with Anna. "You two always work things out," she would say to me.

Once when I was involved with another woman and we broke up, I drove in tears to see Bess. She comforted me, explained the other woman to me, why it was hopeless to begin with. I kept having adventures and kept going to Bess to tell her about them. She would reassure me, and make me feel that she liked me, that I was special, that I'd be okay.

My relationship with her clearly provided me with a base of emotional reassurance. Still I often felt it was flat or dull, and so I tried to prick it, to make it feel more alive, to get Bess to respond to me more, and she would often stop me. Our relationship often felt furtive to me. The complexity of it was hidden, as if such depth was not supposed to be there. Perhaps the hiddenness made my feelings last longer, made Bess into a silent lingering presence that is still so strongly with me. I still talk to her sometimes in my mind as if I really could, as if I will see her soon again, walk into that quiet darkened living room and tell her all my news.

Now in the restaurant, I wanted to go to her. I wanted Bess's white-haired glow to be cast on me. I wanted her to look at me and smile at me as she used to. I wanted her affectionate holding of me even amidst all the awkwardness I expected she would feel. I wanted a sense of lost love found, of this other embrace from a time in my past I had never wanted to leave. For something was aroused in me back then, and more importantly, recognized as legitimate—my need for mothering and protection. This need was a vulnerability I had always before felt had to be kept secret, but I now found it could bring others close to me. Bess came close, as did Anna. That then they found they had needs of their own led to difficulties and to questions in my mind about who was offering what, whose needs were being met, whose denied? How much was I, a receiver of Bess's care, also a giver to her of care? Why were my needs for mothering so strangely mixed with sexual desire? Would they always be so mixed? Would other women draw back from me because of my needs?

I left New Mexico at the end of my second year for a position at a university in California, but in subsequent years, I kept returning on visits as if to find an embrace I had lost. On my visits, I sought to recapture the warmth I had once felt but not the pain, the closeness but not the loneliness. I traveled around looking at the countryside, seeking to find, in the shapes of hills and land, a substitute for an emotional landscape I had once known, a fulfillment of promises once made to me that here I would be cherished and feel I had a home.

Now, however, I feared I would be received harshly if I went up to Bess. She might speak sarcastically to me or act remote because I had left. When I moved away, I left her, and she then left me, although at the time I did not realize the finality of my leaving. When I came back to visit two years later, bringing Hannah, whom I had met in California, we stayed with Bess and Marie in a new house they had moved to near the river. Bess let me know on that visit that her life had gone on without me. "I won't be here for you anymore," she kept telling me by her actions. She cancelled dates to have dinner and withdrew in the kitchen when I came up to touch her. I went to her in her bedroom one night, seeking to arouse her desire, but she pulled away and shook her head. "Why are you treating me like a motel?" she asked me. I was hurt. I had not known I was doing that. I was aware only of my own broken heart.

I next saw her several years later on a visit, but it was much the same. On that trip, Hannah and I went out to dinner with Bess and Marie one night, and Bess acted like she hardly knew me. On our current trip, I did not plan to see her, but I thought of her often and I missed her. When staying in town, Hannah and I often drove past where Bess's new house was located, but I did not remember the exact address, so I kept looking out for it when we were nearby. I looked for a yellow Volvo parked in a driveway. Bess had bought the yellow Volvo after she sold her white Ford pickup. (The cars of people of my past always stay in my mind and seem to stand for the people. I remember the exact models and colors of the cars, which are easier for me to remember than a person's face.) After driving by several times, it seemed to me that a gray concrete wall now stood in front of the house where Bess had lived. I soon began to sense that she no longer lived there. I looked in the phone book for her address but could not find her name. I looked for Marie's name and found someone with her last name listed in an adjoining town.

"So they moved," I thought. It made sense. Marie had probably retired from her job; she was older than Bess. Bess probably drove into the city for her job. Probably it was cheaper to live out there. Maybe Bess had felt their house in town was too noisy and so they had built the wall, or maybe the people who moved in after them had built the wall. I was clearly making things up, making up the connections so an absence would become a presence, so I would know where Bess was and not feel her gone.

Standing now in the Mexican restaurant behind the wooden post, I talked with Hannah about whether to go up to the woman with the silver hair and say hello. "You'll get hurt," Hannah said. "There is a difference between what you wish will happen and what really will happen." Reluctantly, I left without going up to Bess. I do not think she saw me. I walked out of the restaurant with Hannah, into the night, and across the street to where we had parked our car. I looked for Bess's yellow Volvo in the lot among the other cars. Not finding it, I decided she now had a gray Saab. It seemed the most likely of the cars there. Only then did I remember that this restaurant was one that, long ago, Bess had mentioned to me. It was the kind of place she and Marie ate at—nondescript food, old-fashioned, fairly empty. It must have been her I saw, I thought, although I still was not sure it was Marie. Hannah and I drove to another restaurant nearby that had more people in it and better food and we ate dinner. We sat at a blue formica-topped table under bright lights. I looked out the window at the cars passing by in the darkness on the highway. Just past that highway, take another turn. That's where Bess was, I kept thinking.

Sitting across the table from Hannah, I felt shaken, excited, and still shocked by what I had seen. I felt I had seen my past and not gone up to it. I felt warmed by having seen Bess. I told myself she was on her way home from farther north to the town where she now lived near Albuquerque. I could not believe she lived around here; it was too far from where she had lived when I knew her. What had happened? I thought. Why didn't Bess still like me? Why was Marie's hair not also gray? How could Bess seem so close, so much the woman I knew, yet I could not go up to her? I could not reach out and touch her. I was afraid of being seen and hurt. Why did I have to get hurt? Why are my relationships with the women of my past so often like this?

Why are lesbian relationships like this? They extend beyond a couple into threesomes and more broadly and link up unlikely people with one another. They are irregular when looked at closely. They provide a temporary outer balance for an uncertain inner life. They are full of attempts by women to be more to each other than anyone expects—"I will help you. I will be better to you than any-one else has been," we repeatedly tell each other.

Lesbian relationships linger long after the need for them seems gone. They are beneath the surface, often invisible and often viewed as illicit. They are tempting, in part, because they are forbidden. They are like a subterranean world glimpsed only sometimes in pass-ing in the night, like a woman seen in the dark in a Mexican restau-rant who sits across from another woman of unknown relation to her, and who seems like someone I knew very well a long time ago.

"I'm jealous," Hannah said, as we sat in the restaurant. "I'm afraid this will take you over and you won't be here with me."

"You don't need to be afraid," I told her. "That was my past. I don't want to be with her anymore." How simple that is to say, how much harder to believe.

I am still shaken when I think of that experience. I believe I saw Bess. I find it hard to believe I walked out, that I broke a tie with someone important to me. The image of Bess in the restaurant is so clear to me in my mind. I did not expect to see her there, or to see anyone I knew. I had thought I was alone. I had thought I could go to places of my past without seeing the people of my past.

I am still surprised that I did not approach Bess. I preferred to surround her in my mind with a halo of emotions, some of them warm, some of them difficult and unforgiving. Why not me? I wanted to ask her. Why not forever?

In the years that have passed since I left New Mexico, since I stopped living in the desert, I have had many dreams in which I re-turn to a building that, when I wake and decipher it, is Bess and Marie's house. In these dreams, I look for Bess and cannot find her. She has left me, or keeps leaving me. In one of the dreams, her house had black wrought-iron grillwork inside, like the bars on the Mexi-can restaurant. Once it was a shopping center. Once it was a spiritual retreat with pillows on the floor, which was reached at the end of a very long hall that had no walls. In none of the dreams have I ever seen Bess. She is always invisible in the background, and I am always seeking her.

When I lived nearby and knew her, I thought that my relationship with Bess was less deep for me than my other relationship at the time, with Anna. I never expected that my tie to Bess would end up carrying so much weight in my life that it has come to stand for "home" in my dreams. It is the home I have always sought and never found, the home it was not, rather than the home it was. Why this twist? What was the emotional reality back then? What is it now? Why do I embroider my past and seek, in it, a haven, a sense of the world that is mine? Why do I attach my dreams to my past and think it is better than my present can ever be?

I know only that when I walked out of the Mexican restaurant, I felt I had found what I came for. I had glimpsed a reality that once was important to me that was now made all the more present by seeing Bess's familiar face. I see her still in my mind in the living room of that small adobe house set back behind the earthen wall. She is reading in her chair. She gets up from her chair to go meet me at the door. She smiles as she opens the door and holds it for me. I step inside. The lamp is on beside the couch near the doorway that leads to the kitchen. That part of the room is quite warm. We go over to the couch hand-in-hand and sit down. "I saw you in the restaurant," I tell her. "I know," she answers, and we sit and talk and touch, and there are no impossible silences, no strict line is between us. I feel involved, alive, protected, comforted.

SEVEN

Lesbophobia

In this chapter, I describe some very personal images, scenes, and experiences that help me understand why lesbianism so often becomes invisible. I hope that by focusing on my own inner fears I can contribute to the lessening of such fears, for they are all the more effective to the extent they are unacknowledged.

WHEN I THINK ABOUT MY FEARS of lesbianism, my first image is of walking down the street and having small children call after me, taunting me. I live in San Francisco and you would not expect this to be a problem here as much as in other places, but I wonder if the difference is exaggerated. Once, not long ago, I walked down a street and a young girl who must have been about twelve called after me, "Sweet or sour? Sweet or sour?" Then she turned to a small boy walking with her who looked about eight and said to him, "sour." Once, my lover and I were a block from our house, and a girl at a bus stop, also with a young boy, called after us repeatedly, "Are you two men? Are you two men?" until we answered. I have walked along and had young boys in their early teens jump out of entryways to

78

buildings or dart out from bus stops calling "dyke" at me, then turn their heads and run away. I recently walked past a group of boys on a sidewalk near my home who called at me "bull dagger" as I passed. At a beach just north of San Francisco, at a remote bridge leading across a lagoon near the ocean, my lover and I were returning from a walk along the shore when a very young boy, perhaps age four, was arriving with his mother. He was coming over the bridge following her. Repeatedly, he called out to us, "Why are you dressed the same? Why are you dressed the same?" I did not feel we looked so much the same as that we did not look like his mother. No skirt, no blousy shirt. We were not straight women.

I fear walking down the street, because I look like a lesbian. I fear having my lover touch me or hold hands. I fear, and I am convinced my fear is realistic, that someone, some young kid, probably a boy, will pull out a gun and shoot me, or us. I do not want to find out that my fears are valid through harsh experience.

When the repeated taunters are young children, I have wondered why. I have thought that in some way the fears and assaults aimed at me because I am a lesbian have been passed down to these children by their parents. I have noticed how the taunts are most often indirect, not "you fucking queer," or "dyke," but "Hey men," or "You're ugly," or comments on our clothes. I have noticed how I get more taunts when there are two of us. I have noted that except on one occasion, I have never taunted back. I am too afraid of the hidden gun, too afraid of the public exposure, the open street. The one time I did speak back to a taunting child was to the girl who called "sweet or sour." After I had listened carefully for two blocks to make sure I got the drift of her indirect taunt, I walked over and said to her, "Are you afraid of lesbians? Are you afraid of being one? Do you want to be close with women? Who makes you afraid?" She quickly ducked into a nearby corner store, afraid now of me. I was unnerved. I did not enjoy intimidating a child, taunting back. I would rather go on in silence, rather absorb it. I felt sure she did not understand. I felt that on a street corner, for the time I had of less than a minute, I could not convince her, or show her. For the underlying feelings, like the taunts, are indirect, cross-wired, balled up. When I asked, "Are you afraid of being a lesbian? Are you afraid of being like me?" she would have no way of understanding what I meant.

Not long ago, three older teenaged boys taunted me. They were sitting on a flight of steps beside a small park. I was walking up the steps past them."Stone cold, stone cold," they murmured loud enough for me to hear. I turned, "What do you mean?" I asked. "It's a phrase from wrestling," the larger one said. "Don't you know it? Do you follow wrestling? Stone cold? Stone cold." "No," I said, as if dumb, as if it made no sense, and I walked on up the steps. But it had made eminent sense to me, the indirectness of their taunt. "Stone cold," I felt, meant stone butch. I am used to this. Often I feel I would prefer the directness, though not the gun.

A few years ago when my book *The Family Silver* came out, I had planned to go on a speaking tour. After giving two initial talks, however, I felt too exposed. I found it too difficult speaking personally about my inner lesbian experiences to strangers in a lecture hall or seminar room who would afterward change the subject to gay men, to general prejudices people had in Iowa where, of course, it was much worse than here in a university. And I, who had just explained why it was hard for me in a university, would wonder why they had to say this. I would feel hurt because in a room full of women, the question askers would almost all be men, talking about themselves. It was one thing for me to write a personal book in which I spoke of my lesbianism, an intimate fact, an intimate inner experience of huge definitional weight in my life; it was one thing to write about this, another to stand before others and speak of it and hear what they would say back.

I was mindful, too, of the fact that the book I was withdrawing from speaking about was called *The Family Silver: Essays on Relationships among Women,* rather than *The Family Silver: Essays on Lesbian Relationships,* or something with lesbian in the title. This was my fourth published book, but like the others, the word *lesbian* was noticeably absent. When I looked back and realized this omission, I felt like such a coward. I did not notice it until near publication, when I saw the table of contents for the book in the final page proofs and realized how many chapter titles contained the word lesbian, or a euphemism for it. Initially, I had been critical when publishers sent my manuscript out to lesbian reviewers. Why do that? I thought. Why see it as a lesbian book? Why not a women's book? Why sexualize it? That's what people always do to lesbians.

Then when the first newspaper review of my book came out and spoke of it as a lesbian book—it was about a lesbian professor, the reviewer said, about "lesbian family silver"—I felt proud, acknowledged. This was how I wanted to be seen. Yet I could not announce it in my title. I still feared that word lesbian. The "s" and "b" together looked to me so round and soft. This word has always reminded me of myself when I was a round, soft "chubby" child, the child I felt others took a distance from—because of my chubbiness, because of my lesbianism? Definitely because of my inner needs for nurturance, for maternal caring. Are these separate?

I had previously written a book about a lesbian community and it, too, did not have lesbian in the title. I was afraid it would be put on a lesbian shelf and no one would read it, a fear I still have. I am writing a new book now, and I am struggling with what to do about the word *lesbian*. I take it out, for I have a hard time putting it in my title in any way that seems acceptable to me. I fear it will limit my book; it would not seem to be about anything that anyone but lesbians would read. It simply looks awkward. They won't understand. I will be rejected. I'll be dead.

For five years I taught a course on lesbian communities and identities. The class was always very small; the largest, four students the first year. Twice I had only one student. Most of the students who turned out for the first class session each year to consider the course were not lesbian, and at least half who took it over the years were not lesbian, although they were all women. Those who were lesbian did not want to use the word to refer to themselves and spent much of the quarter struggling with that. I pushed them—I said, why avoid it? what does it mean? what are you afraid of?—knowing my own fears. In the end, those struggling began to use the word, to risk, to dare. But by the end of each term, actually after the first two weeks, the classes became smaller. Those afraid of a teacher who encouraged the word *lesbian,* who viewed them also as afraid, left for other classes that were more "interesting," or because of a "heavy workload," some promising to come back next year, but they never did. So my classes would go from four to two, from two to one.

At the time I taught my lesbian course, from the very first year when I had a class of four women—one lesbian, three not—I found I had to deal with two subjects all the time: fears of lesbianism, which I called "lesbophobia," to distinguish it from fears of gay male sexuality or of homosexuality more generally, and lesbianism itself. I learned to tell the students that we had to deal with both subjects because their and my fears repeatedly got in the way of understanding lesbianism for what it was. Our fears prevented us from seeing it clearly and caused us to retreat from it. I also learned to expect "acting out" in my classes—students coming late, coming barefoot, arguing with me, bringing lesbian friends who would be critical, telling me things that did not, on the surface, make sense to me. The students would do assignments incompletely, be easily hurt, easily angry, strike out in a passive-aggressive manner.

Still, my lesbian course went well despite the odd behaviors, and each year we reached important insights and were close in the end. But after five years of teaching the course, when, for the second time, I had only one student, I decided not to offer it the next year, and perhaps never again. No one strictly told me, "you can't go on doing this." However, I knew I could not continue to teach a course to which no one came. There had been one student this year, but next year there might not be any; having one student was awfully close to having none. So I shut myself down, before someone else did. I had always felt others were going to come and wipe me out, so I did it first. I always felt it was my fault the enrollment was tiny and I feared it would reflect badly upon me. Still, I was angry at them—at all those who believed the university was liberal, that people were more accepting now. "But they would not take my course," I wanted to say. "The students would not support it, they would not support me."

That last year of my lesbian course, a graduate student who had been initially interested called me the first week. "I can't take it," she said. "My career." I felt hurt and abandoned. I tried to argue with her but felt I should not. That year, the student who took the course and I walked around the campus all quarter angry each time we saw a woman who looked like a lesbian. Why wasn't she in our class? What was wrong with her? What was wrong with us? "Maybe if the university offered to pay them to take the course, maybe they'd do it," the one student said. "Then maybe they'd give a donation later." "Maybe if I changed the name," I thought, "if I took *lesbian* out of the title, or put it last." "But that's what I looked for in the course listings," she said, "the word, anything with the word." "Why am I the only one?" this student asked. We shared the aloneness.

As a result of teaching my lesbian course, I began to include more lesbian readings in my other classes. I found them interesting and they helped me teach some important lessons, especially about the presence of lesbophobia within each of us. I also thought that if the students read more it might ease tensions I had always felt as a lesbian teacher. Yet I found that as soon as I gave lesbianism more attention in my classes, the students struck out more—as had the kids on the street—though indirectly. They would challenge an assignment or something I said. "Why aren't we talking about 'biphobia'?" one would say when I asked them to talk about lesbophobia. "Because it's not about lesbianism, the subject is lesbianism." Or a student would call out angrily at me after doing a reading, "But what about me? What about straight women?" A student might speak negatively of an assignment, "I think it's dangerous. I don't want to do it." I was surprised, since I was used to thinking of my assignments as helpful, not dangerous. I now had to think about what was being feared.

Along with introducing the lesbian materials, I would ask the students to see lesbianism as a choice, or to see how it could be a choice, or a product of culture, rather than a result of biology. They would push me away. "I don't believe that," even a lesbian student would say. When I assigned readings that included discussions of lesbian sex, the students would often turn the subject to their boyfriends and heterosexual sex. At first, I was surprised. Then I began to notice the "changing of the subject" that often occurred when I introduced a lesbian topic. The students turned to heterosexuality, to the sensitivities of straight women, or of queer or bisexual women, or of men. Even lesbian students would do this, as if protecting others from themselves.

The more I used lesbian material, the more I found that lesbian students would disagree with me in my classes, especially when discussing a lesbian topic, as if they needed to make clear that they were different from me. They would not use the word *lesbian* if I did, for example, or they would disagree with me when I asserted that discrimination against lesbians still existed. Their distance made me feel I was the only lesbian in the room.

At times it seemed that group solidarity was accomplished in my classes by the students excluding me—leaving me at break time, abandoning my points in discussions of lesbian issues, treating me as if I was a "lesbian threat." I felt that in their eyes I was perhaps a stereotypical "big bad lesbian" who they expected would seduce and reject them. Perhaps because lesbianism is so sexualized, they saw me in the bedroom and wanted to be intimately loved and accepted by me. But because I was also a teacher in a classroom, giving assignments and having requirements, a student could easily feel hurt or rejected by any accidental harshness. The student might then strike out, rejecting me first. One year, at the start of the term, I told the students, "I don't want to be seen as your mother, and I don't want to be seen as the 'big bad lesbian' who is going to hurt you." But, I thought, how could they understand it?

I knew that the students in my lesbian course had feared inter-viewing lesbians, which was one of my assignments. They feared les-bians would reject them for not measuring up to the expectations lesbians had of them. If they feared other lesbians, probably they feared me. I felt I had to step carefully, and not overwhelm them with who I was.

The final year of my lesbian course, knowing that it would soon end, I was especially intent on teaching about lesbianism in my other course at the time, a feminist research class that consisted en-tirely of women. Yet the more I tried to teach about lesbianism, the more I felt the students easily became reactive. I felt they needed my caring, and in a way my self-obliteration, as if in compensation for the stereotype of the unforgiving lesbian, the lesbian who punishes straight women for being straight and lesbians for not being lesbian enough. I was perhaps particularly sensitive that quarter because I was feeling the loss of my lesbian class.

The turning point for me was a moment midway through the term when I told the students I thought lesbianism was a choice, that there was a "lesbian/straight" divide, and that it made a differ-ence if one was on the lesbian side of it. The students became unset-tled. They did not want to be divided from one another or from me. They wanted not to have to make a choice. They came to my office, some quite disturbed, and asked me, "What about our relation-ship?" Would I still love them? Did I care about them? They needed to know it was okay with me if they were straight, that I approved of their sleeping with men, or if they were lesbian, of their disagreeing with me. And here was the difficulty for me, the provocative threat: they needed to tell me they felt our class dynamics had taken a sud-den bad turn and I had to do something or else the class would fall apart. I cared about my class. I told the students, "It's okay with me if you are straight. It's okay if you don't agree with me. Yes, these are just my own thoughts."

After I apologized for saying things distressing to them and smoothed things over, the students felt better and the course worked out well in the end. However, I knew I had felt rejected. As the quarter drew to a close, I withdrew increasingly, feeling hurt, and I hid my lesbianism far more than I wanted to. I felt that the students had taken me for granted. They seemed to want lesbian inclusion—the benefits of being a lesbian, of being nurtured by a lesbian teacher—without the risks, without the affiliations. They wanted the benefits without being one. Yet by the end of the term, I, too, had taken steps toward invisibility because of my fears. Still, I hoped that the feelings raised as a result of exposure to a lesbian emotional landscape would be instructive in the long run, for all of us. Perhaps the next time, there would be less pulling away.

When I think about effects of lesbophobia on my teaching, I am reminded of certain moments from my past. Once years ago, I went out to dinner with a woman I was getting to know who was clearly straight, a nurse, a sweet woman. As we sat in a red-vinyl booth in a restaurant, she looked over at me and said, as if it were quite natural, "I don't want to go to bed with you." Had I asked? I thought. Had I done something? "Of course," I nodded, "I understand that." I did not say, "I don't want to go to bed with you either." She seemed relieved. Something important had been clarified. However, I felt hurt. Was I so awful as to need to be rejected beforehand? Why did I have to agree that, of course, she would not want to go to bed with me? Perhaps she should want to. It might be a good experience. Or did she want to? Was I being rejected because I was seductive? Had I been seductive? Our relationship never was the same again, because of this sour note, this closed possibility. And I saw myself again as the chubby child who, as a lesbian, was being pushed away. No one would want me.

During the same period, I spent a night with another woman who I believed was straight and who was somewhat seductive. Why do I fall for straight women, for the mother, the figure of female nurturance? After dinner in her home, we sat close together on the couch. She lay beside me and we talked quietly. Then we moved to her bed, where she lay back and I touched her. But she seemed suddenly cold and stiff, as if waiting for me to soften her, loosen her, make her feel as only a lesbian can. I felt on trial, tested to prove I could overcome and correct for all the past hurts in her life. I felt the power of my role: of what was assigned to me, my supposed gifts. I sat back. I did not want this job. I did not want to have to prove I was worth it. I did not want to save her. Feeling resentful, I pulled away and soon left. I will always remember the fear in her eyes, the cold stillness, the waiting. It is the same remote fear I sense in the students.

Yet I know that lesbian sex can raise past hurts for me, too. I often draw back rather than open up or relax. Even with my lover of nineteen years, though we take care with each other and have sweet loving times together in bed, old hurts can arise for me. There is something very vulnerable, very unreal, very exposed in lesbianism. I want the ideal. I want my lover to hold me as a child, touch me, surround me, make me forget the world outside. I want her gentle touch, the feeling of her body as my safety. Yet I consciously struggle to feel safe each time, to feel the bedroom is safe, our bedroom. The walls to the outside feel too thin, the neighbors too near. My lesbianism emphasizes my fears. It makes me afraid to find out that I am unprotected, afraid to be open, afraid to feel safe. It causes me constantly to invent, to surround myself and my lover with something that will make me feel we are protected.

The fears that come with lesbianism clearly permeate my intimacies. They do not stop at any bedroom door. Although lesbian sex is often discussed as if it were purely pleasure and safe haven, I think what is overlooked is that in lesbian intimacies especially, fears and old hurts can arise acutely. It takes figuring out ways to deal with them, ways not to withdraw, and not to reproduce heterosexuality in the face of the fears, but rather to find something new.

"When will the vulnerability end?" a student once asked me. She was newly a lesbian. She also asked, "Is it worth it? You have to tell me again and again that it is." I did not entirely understand her request, so often do I tuck away my own fears.

Why is lesbianism so frightening? I know that for me it is frightening to depend on another woman. It raises my inner needs for nurturance and love from my mother, who had her own problems, and who could not always respond well, who as a woman herself had been wounded, who could not be the ideal. To be a lesbian raises my fears of female vulnerability and my desires to have my deepest needs met. It raises desires for a perfect healing from an imperfect source, another woman, who, too, is afraid, and who, too, has been hurt.

If heterosexuality is somehow completion of a female-male bond, lesbianism is perhaps an incompletion—a desire for perfection, for the perfect happiness, the perfect safety and freedom. It is a very different dream from heterosexuality, and I am never done learning about it.

When I was first a lesbian and began living with a woman lover, her first lesbian lover, from twenty years before, came to visit us one night. She brought her current young lover. After dinner, the four of us were sitting around in the living room talking. The light was low, the feeling comfortable. My lover's former lover, now aged sixty, turned to me and asked, as if welcoming me into a private club, "What do you think of the lesbian lifestyle?" "What lifestyle?" I threw back at her. "I don't think there is one." I was in my mind focused on the fact that there were many. I was not wanting to think about lesbianism. I was only newly one. I did not want to be identified. I did not want to answer her question, as my students often do not want to answer mine—Why are you afraid of being a lesbian? Why are you afraid of the word? I was being indirect, as are the kids on the street. I made it seem as if this were a matter of thought, as if I disagreed with this woman, this older lesbian who, in her own indirect way, was welcoming me in. She was saying, "Here come and sit beside me, it is safe. There is something bigger going on. You are not just alone. It's a world."

Back then, I could not accept the invitation. I did not want to be like this woman. I wanted to be young and free, to make up my own mind, to see it my own way. I wanted to be alone. I still do. And now I am older; the time has flown by, yet much remains the same. I want to welcome others in, yet I am afraid to. I have my own indirectness. I go it alone. Yet I am more aware now, and in a way more humble, more angry, and less brave. When I was first a lesbian, I felt proud to touch my lover in public and to put my arm around her when walking down the street. However, I no longer feel so safe. Perhaps the world is less safe, or perhaps I have come to feel less safe because I know more. I have my own battle scars. I have experienced the degree of my own vulnerability.

I now have my life so deeply vested in lesbianism, so much depends on it for me. The question of respect is more serious. I want no taunts, no ungrateful children. I want recognition, appreciation. I have had enough slights, and enough invisibility—as when I stand with my lover in an airport talking; we look meaningfully at each other, and people, usually men, walk right through us. Or when I sit in a classroom and bring up the subject of lesbianism and students look past it and me.

As a lesbian, I feel I represent an ideal of what women can give to each other. At the same time, I confront fears of that ideal—on the streets, in the classroom, in bed with other women, in conversations over dinner. I am often hurt by these fears. When I am called a name, or oddly questioned, or when I feel rejected, I may withdraw because of my sensitivities. Yet I need to remind myself to hold fast to my own inner vision that says that the fears I sense are real, tangible, important, no matter how often they masquerade as something else, or seem not to be there. If I doubt their power, I need only look within myself. The invisible landscape of lesbianism is also a landscape of invisible fears.

PART 3

Blindness and Sight

EIGHT

Losing My Vision

This chapter introduces a series on losing my eyesight. In it, I reflect on the nature of vision—what it is, how it can be maintained, and how unique inner visions can be valued. Just as the geographic landscapes described in earlier chapters had changed when I revisited them, so too, when I began to lose my eyesight, the outer world literally became no longer visible to me as it had been before. I soon began to create a counterposing internal vision so that my sense of my own value would remain intact. I think we are all to some extent blind, to some extent sighted, and each of us moves in a world of unique inner vision, an interior landscape that is composed of meanings, of sights and sounds, and feelings deeply held.

I AM LOSING MY EYESIGHT. I am not sure if my vision loss will continue for a few years more or indefinitely. Already my visual world has changed. I no longer see clearly objects at a distance—trees, buildings, street signs. There are many things I simply do not see—small lines, light colors on light backgrounds. In the mid-distance,

93

the definition in people's faces disappears, as do the titles of books on shelves a few feet from me. I need magnifiers to read, or I need to enlarge the print using a computer printer or a large screen because normal-sized print looks tiny to me.

Objects that move quickly into my peripheral vision often hit a blind spot and then suddenly appear before me, startling me. These might include a car pulling away from a curb, a person coming into a room from my side, a grocery bag at my feet, an open cabinet door. I will step on the bag and bump into the cabinet door because I do not see them. I have gotten used to bumping into things and to scanning from left to right when I drive or when I enter a room looking for my baseball hat or my pen or a glass I have left on a surface somewhere.

I look very carefully at objects directly in front of me so that I will cut them or move them properly—so I can cut carrots without cutting my hand, or put a pen into its cap without missing the hole. Sometimes I will not see a glass on a table because I see right through it; I do not see the edges. Similarly, I have to be careful on stairs because the edges are not clear to me.

In low or less than bright light, I will not see details or colors well. I will misdial a phone number because I do not see the markings on the key pads; I will not appreciate fully the color of a shirt I am wearing. I find I often stare intently at the controls on the washing machine in my basement, trying to turn the knob to the proper setting. At night in the dark, I will not see the edges of a path I am walking on and so I may lose my way; I have to shine a flashlight on my black dog when I am walking him in order to see him. I am always reaching for flashlights and lighted magnifiers and turning on all the lamps in a room so I will be comfortable and better able to see.

Sometimes it will take a while, even in broad daylight, for an image to compose itself in front of me so I can know what it is—is that a truck in my view a half block away, for instance, or a building against the sky? Recently when my lover and I were visiting a house for sale in the neighborhood, she bumped her head into a low doorway when coming in from the yard, fell down, and called to me to help her. From a distance, I thought she was a garbage can overturned and lying on the ground. I saw a man down the street with a parrot on his shoulder who turned out to be a woman with a pony tail. While driving on the highway in the rain, I saw a monster shaped like a dinosaur emerge from the mist by the roadside. It was a highway exit sign. Each of these misperceptions has disturbed me because I did not see something for what it was.

I no longer take my vision for granted. During the past year, my vision has changed for the worse in ways I notice about once every two months. As a result, I am very aware that what I see now is a temporary state. I often feel sad about what is happening to my vision. But my major problem is not that I focus on what I no longer see, but that I fear that in the future I will not be able to see what I see now, blurred as it is. I worry, what will happen to me when my vision gets worse? What if I can't see at all? What if I can't read, can't clean house, can't write, can't drive, can't walk distances as I do now looking around and appreciating the scenery?

What if I can't see the flowers in my yard or the plants I am trying to grow, or take care of my pets? What if the colors disappear and the flowers that now look blurred to me no longer have any color? Several years ago, I took up birdwatching. What if I can no longer see the birds? Already, their outlines and colored markings look broken to me when I view them through my binoculars. What if my appearance gets bad because I cannot see myself well enough? What if I begin to wear pink and no longer look like myself or like a lesbian? What if people feel uncomfortable around me and have no use for me because I cannot see them? Will I get mugged on the street? Will people patronize me?

Sometimes I just want to close my eyes and go blind suddenly so that I will know what it will be like and that I will be okay.

It was only a year ago that my vision became much worse than it had been. During the two previous years, I had noticed dark floaters in front of my eyes, small round disks that covered the blue sky with what looked like fine splattered drops of mud. The print on the page had become small. But last spring, the changes in my vision became more pronounced. I noticed that the grills on the cars and trucks suddenly looked wavy and irregular, and like they had chunks taken out of them. This made the cars look smashed in. Soon the letters on street signs also looked like they had chunks taken out. It looked to me like all the straight lines around me had acid thrown on them or like they were dissolving under water. Telephone poles, power lines, edges of windows and doors on houses, lines marking crosswalks and the lanes on highways all looked bent and as if parts of them were dissolving away.

I was very upset by what I was seeing. The outer world looked to me like it had been in an accident, or car wreck. What I saw outside, I felt, was happening to my eyes. Sometimes I thought they, too, had acid thrown on them, although they did not hurt me. I felt damaged and very alone, and as if I were walking around in an unusual and partly destroyed external world, seeing what no one else was seeing.

Two kinds of changes that started last spring affected me most of all. First was reading. Increasingly, the print on the page looked small and bent and the letters looked like they had bites taken out of them. They looked as if they were under water and had many dark cobweb shapes floating around on top of them. I found that I could not read except with strong magnifiers. With these magnifiers, I could read only a few words at a time; my reading became very slow; I could not scan; I started to cry. Without the magnifiers, I could not read labels on packages, signs in supermarkets, street signs unless I was right under them, my own handwriting unless I wrote big and dark. I could not walk into a bookstore and browse or keep up with the new books. The thought of reading an entire book seemed an immensely large undertaking. I felt my reading world was slipping away.

I had not realized before how important reading was to me. It was one thing for the grills on the cars to look smashed in, but I feared that not reading meant I would not be able to have an inner world. I would not be able to bring in information and to nourish myself and create a world I could be in even if I could not see.

In addition, my main work is writing. It has always depended upon my seeing words and phrases in front of me so I can know how to revise them. I type and retype my pages many times, reading them over using a visual aesthetic that is very connected to a voice in my head. This inner written voice is different from my spoken voice. As my reading became difficult, I worried, what would happen if I could no longer see my writing? I felt I would lose my ability to do it.

Looking at the cracked letters on my pages and in books by others made me sad. The breaking of these letters seemed to represent more destructiveness than when the cars looked smashed in.

The second change that made me cry was the blurring away of people's faces—the fading out of the details of features, skin tones, and facial outlines. When walking down the street, I noticed I was seeing the clothes and forms of people, but their faces looked bleached out, so I stared at the faces trying to make out what they looked like. I found that people then said hello to me, as if they thought I knew them, embarrassing me. I told myself to look down quickly, because people usually avert their gaze from strangers on the street.

Even from the distance of across a room, as at a party, or across a seminar table when teaching, I found that people's faces looked washed out or in shadow, their features small dark spots. In classes, moving hairlike floaters passing over the students' faces blocked out parts of them. If light came from behind a person, as when a friend sat across from me in my living room with a bright window behind her, her face would turn totally dark. I would try to reposition myself so the light came from behind me. I did not like the feeling of not being able to see someone with whom I was talking.

I noticed that at a distance on the street, the outlines of people's faces sometimes looked geometric and two-part, as if the top of the face was separate from the bottom, and the bottom was a triangle set off to one side. The outlines looked like they had chunks taken out of them, as had the cars and letters; the facial features looked smashed in. I was frightened by the grotesqueness I was seeing.

But most of all, I was upset that increasingly I could not see clearly the faces of people closest to me, whom I usually see from just a few feet away. I was glad one day when at the beach with my lover Hannah, sitting two inches from her in bright sunlight, I was able to see clearly that she had wrinkles. Usually at home, her face will look in shadow to me even across the dining table, and I cannot see the expression or light in her eyes that I am used to. Sometimes I have looked in the mirror at my own face and felt horrified knowing I am not seeing all that is there. Do I have eyebrows? Do my eyes truly look so hollow? What do I really look like? I wonder. What do others see when they look at me?

These changes in what I see continue. I have become used to many of them. I am learning to walk around in a world where people have little definition in their faces. I am learning, even with those close to me, to talk to a blur in the distance, although I do try to get as close as I can most of the time and to turn lights on. I want to see the faces of people I know for as long as I can. Generally I have to remind myself to see as much as I can, to use my eyesight, to drive when I safely can, to plant the flowers I want to see grow, to find ways to read. I have to remind myself to stay in the present where I can deal with things, rather than in the future where I simply have fears.

The eye condition I have is called "birdshot retinochoroidopathy." It is an inflammation in the back of my eyes that started three years ago. I first noticed it when I began to see increasing numbers of floaters—those small dark circles and cobweb shapes spinning before my eyes that caused white pages and light backgrounds to look dirty. The condition began as an inflammation of my choroid—the thin layer of blood vessels that nourish my retina. Then it spread to my retina, affecting both my peripheral, or side, vision and my central vision—the cells which enable me to see fine lines, colors, and details. None of what is affecting my vision is visible to people looking at me normally. An eye doctor has to dilate my pupils and look through them into the backs of my eyes with bright lights in order to see the inflammation and its effects. The condition is called "birdshot" because the scattered lesions in my eyes are said to look like a spray of birdshot from a gun.

My eye condition is a rare disease and is considered to be a result of autoimmune processes. It may flare up and subside at intervals, but it is worrisome because it causes cumulative damage to my eyes over time. The retina has been likened to the film in a camera; when light hits it, it registers an image, transmitted to the brain via the optic nerve. When the inner architecture of the eyes is disturbed—in my case because of swelling and because the sensitive receptor cells (the rods and cones) have been inflamed—the outer images are also changed. I see odd effects, such as those I first noticed last spring when the grills on the cars began to look bent and people's faces started looking blurred and washed out, and when the print on the pages appeared increasingly broken and small.

The changes I started noticing last spring jolted and frightened me, but they also made me think a great deal about what vision is. Do I see with my eyes, or with my mind? I wondered. When I lose my vision, must I change my vocabulary, eliminating all the words to do with sight? Am I truly disadvantaged with less eyesight, or simply different? When my visual world changes—when I see curved lines instead of straight ones, and faces without fine-line detail; when I mistake a pony tail on a woman's head for a parrot on a man's shoulder, and think a road sign is a prehistoric monster—is what I see now distorted and lacking, or only different? How can I keep from making my vision loss into something that makes me feel I am less valuable as a person? How, too, I have wondered, can I not see myself in the terms of the medical world, in which a loss of eyesight is viewed as a failure? How can I not see myself as a set of failed eyes, but rather as a whole person?

There is no effective treatment for my eye condition. Steroid shots and immunosuppressant drugs have been used, but the condition returns as soon as any treatment is stopped and there are dangerous side-effects.

Thus my situation is both uncertain and frightening. I hold out a hope that miraculously, I will one day get better. I will wake up one morning and my eyes will see well again. I will look in the mirror to put in my earrings and be able to see the small holes where the posts should go. I will see Hannah's face clearly. I will no longer have to grasp bannisters tightly when I walk down steps. I will be able to read unaided. The world will again be full of true vivid colors and much clarity of definition. But I must expect not to see that well again, because mine is most likely a chronic and progressive condition.

My eye doctor, a retinal specialist whom I like, once told me that "my birdshot" would eventually burn itself out. It was a question of how much of my vision it would take with it. At a later time, he told me he thought the condition would not burn out in my case. There is that indeterminacy.

There is also the image. When my eye doctor used the word "burn," it made me feel there was a fire in my eyes. It is a painless fire in that my eyes do not hurt inside from the inflammation at the back of them, although sometimes I feel sore externally from straining my muscles in order to see—such as when I drive or read a lot or am tired.

Having an eye condition that causes a loss of vision is something new for me. It is old in that I have had physical difficulties before, such as chronic migraine headaches and arthritis, and I have long struggled with emotional dilemmas that can make life a challenge. My vision loss seems to me similar to those experiences in that I must accommodate it and take it into account in all that I do. It is different in that it seems to me more glaring, more obvious, perhaps easier to understand. It is also different because it is considered by the culture, or larger world, as more serious and more of a loss. I know I feel it as a loss, and I fear it will be a loss, but I also feel it as a change. I feel it puts me into the world of people who have less than normal vision, and it seems to me there will be some comfort for me in that, although as of yet I am still quite alone.

Definitely, my vision loss is a life change for me. I feel I am walking off into a new space, entering into an exciting adventure. I can put a positive face on what I am experiencing, and often I do, but it is also important for me to acknowledge my fears, the destruction in the world that I see visually, and the losses I feel.

When the Point Reyes National Seashore burned several years ago and I went there after the fire, I watched the landscape change. The rolling hills became bright green and clear; new grasses grew, free of the overbrush that had kept the sunlight from them for years. Bare blackened tree trunks stood like sculptures against the sky. Tall yellow flowers tossed about in the wind by the roadside, the sea stretching out looking glassy behind them. There was an exquisite clarity all around me. I saw a different picture than I had before the fire.

I cannot see that same picture at Point Reyes now, both because the external scenery has changed once again—the ground scrub has grown back thicker and duller in color, and the once silhouetted black trees have weathered and turned gray, blending back in—and because my internal vision has changed. The blue irises I now look at in the spring on the hills that slope toward the ocean are blurred; I have to take out my binoculars to see them. I have to take out my binoculars at the beach to see the waves and to see any detail in the white foamy breakers. The large forms and colors of sand dunes and green meadows surround me as I walk on a path toward the beach. I sit in a crevice among the dunes surrounded by scattered clumps of low-lying white flowers, a garden of beauties I can barely see. I am going to have to grow accustomed to this new world I am in—if indeed it keeps being mine—and to find and delight in my place in it.

NINE

Birdwatching before Sunrise

In this portrait of a visit to a desert wildlife refuge, I describe a special time of day—between darkness and morning light—and a particular time in my life, when my eyesight was becoming increasingly uncertain. "Birdwatching before Sunrise" is an adventure in vision, full of the lights, colors, and shapes that surround me as I look out onto a desert landscape with changed sight.

DRIVING IN THE DARK

On a dark, chilly morning that felt like nighttime, I was excited to be off. I woke at 4 a.m., showered, brewed strong coffee, poured it into a thermos, took coffee cake, my binoculars, camera, flashlights, and warm clothes. I stepped carefully through the low-lying, dark country house where I was staying, moving from the kitchen toward the front door, shining my flashlight ahead of me at every step. I did not want to bump into a bookcase or doorway. Outside, I shined my light on the front porch step leading down into the dirt lot beside the house.

The sky overhead was black, the air still. I had to be very careful backing my car up in the lot because I did not want to hit anything in the darkness. A horse whinnied as I moved the car, startling me. She ran off to another part of an adjacent lot that I had seen in the daylight—a lot covered with brambly weeds and, in the center, the thick, brown, roofless walls that had once been an adobe house.

I turned out of the driveway and onto a small street, looking for the edges of the road, which were hard for me to see in the darkness. Then I turned on my brights, looking for the intersection of this small road with another cutting into it that went for a block and led to the two-lane, straight state highway leading south, which in eight miles would take me to a bird sanctuary. For several days, I had been planning how I would drive this road in the dark and reach the bird refuge and wait and watch the light in the sky change from night to day and watch the cranes and geese fly up from an isolated marsh in the middle of the desert.

None of this is unusual. Birdwatchers often get up before sunrise to see the first light and catch glimpses of early morning birds. What was unusual was that on this still November morning, I was losing my eyesight. I could not see well in the dark; I could not see much at all without very bright lights in front of me. Because of my decreased eyesight, I had done a dry run of my route to the marsh several times the day before, figuring out the mileage and what my landmarks would be, where I would fasten my eyes on the road, what I would look for beside the road to tell me where my turnoffs were and whether I had gone too far. I had to be able to find my way even though I could not see well.

Fortunately, there were no other cars on the road this early morning. I liked the feeling of quiet all around me and of everyone asleep as I drove out of town. I felt as if I alone owned the earth, was awake, alive, counted. I did not have to worry about distinguishing myself from anyone else. The town I was driving through was a small New

Mexico town—a group of scattered brown and white houses spread on sandy lots near a river and on small roads stretching out from an intersection of two very straight state highways, the intersection marked by a bar and chileburger restaurant, in front of it a phone and a high hanging traffic light.

I turned left on the state road that headed south as it dipped through town a block from the bar, at a spot where a partly lit church loomed silently out of the darkness. After passing a few houses, the road simply went straight; railroad tracks ran beside it; the area around me opened out. On both sides of the road now were fields, some where horses and cows grazed, others were empty and grown over, or sandy and dotted with green scrub. On my left in the east in the near distance was the Rio Grande, snaking its way south. This was silty river bottomland, spreading out like a flat floodplain. On my right to the west were the Chupadera mountains, massive and brown, feeling almost in arm's reach. That was my view in the daytime—a looming presence of brown mountains, green-tinged sandy fields, yellowing cottonwoods in the near distance lining the river, their gold color signaling the coming of late fall. But at night now, there was nothing, no color, no familiar landmarks, just this dark, almost pitch-black road that I was driving, with black on both sides, black ahead and behind me.

A yellow dotted line ran down the center of the asphalt road, but the painting on it was faint. More clear were the white lines on either side of the road, helpful for me because my car's brights would light them up and if I watched them carefully, they would enable me to stay on the road by showing me where the edges were. Without these lines, it would all be blackness.

I was afraid of the blackness, afraid I would go too fast or too slow. I feared a police car might come get me—the low-vision police who stop people who cannot see. I had trouble reading my car's speedometer. I had to bend my head down and put my eyes close to it to see the markings. When I did so, I worried I might drive off the road. I worried that if a car came from behind me and I was going too slow, it might plow into me; if I went too fast, I might lose control of my car and veer off the road, or into the face of an oncoming car. In the darkness, I might not judge the distance well between myself and another car. I might not be far enough over on my side and so we might collide. I was afraid I would miss my turnoff; I would not reach the marsh, not be able to have the experience I was seeking.

I finally saw the lights of an oncoming car in the far distance, although they seemed close. The car kept coming and coming. The lights seemed big and terribly bright, almost blinding. The road I was driving on was so straight, the morning so dark, that the slightest amount of light was magnified. Then, too, my eye condition exaggerates glare.

The car finally passed. I drove on in the darkness. I looked beside the road in the dark for the landmarks that my lover Hannah, now still safely in bed, had pointed out to me the day before—the railroad crossing that had a bright light above it; the narrow bridge with reflective markers on each side; the spot where a wooden sign stood brown and forestlike next to the road. "You are entering the Bosque del Apache National Wildlife Area," it read, a picture of a flying crane carved beneath the wooden lettering. Then came a stretch where a few houses on a hillside had lights on.

At one point, I thought I saw a rabbit jump out of the roadbed and off into the fields on my side. I was happy I could see something so small, even if it looked like a gray blur.

I felt tense driving. I feared I was driving too fast, although I was going less than the speed limit. My fingers were cold and tight on the steering wheel, my eyes were focused on staying on the road. Finally I saw the small reflective metal sign that told me that my turnoff was coming up, then the second small sign that, were I to pass it, would indicate I had gone too far.

I turned left onto a sandy entry road and into the refuge. Then I passed the square wooden booth where, in the daylight, someone stood to collect fees. In the dark, no one was there. The windows and sides of the booth reflected the light from my car's headlights.

Beyond it, all was dark. Ahead of me in that darkness lay the refuge—a complex of marshes intersected and ringed widely by sandy dirt roads. The marshes were backed by woods and, farther down, by the Rio Grande.

The refuge extended for 57,000 acres. The heart of it, just under one quarter of the total, was low-lying land that was flooded regularly with water from the river to provide feeding and roosting grounds for birds. The marshes in this extensive central basin were made up of ponds and moist fields. At the north end of the refuge were agricultural fields where farmers raised corn for the cranes and geese who came here. Farther out, the refuge lands included desert mesas, arid plains, and portions of the foothills of the nearby mountains. The area, although planned, felt wild. Hundreds of thousands of birds and other animals found sanctuary here in winter. At this time of year, midfall, the arrival of the big birds had already begun. Ahead of me in the marshes, 7,000 sandhill cranes and 17,000 snow geese were now sleeping, or awake but still and making noise.

The sandhill cranes were large gray birds with long necks and a striking red stripe on their heads; they had long legs and a plume of rear gray feathers. They stood out in the dark marshes wading in the watery grasses. The white snow geese, down from the Arctic, were floating out on the shallow marsh ponds along with 38,000 ducks. Other wild birds wintered in the refuge, although less dramatic in number—eagles, cormorants, pheasants, hawks, egrets, owls, kingfishers, avocets, ibis, roadrunners, many songbirds. There were coyotes, mule deer, bobcats, badgers, occasionally a mountain lion. While many birds perched in the trees and brush at night, the sandhill cranes and snow geese spent their nights in the marsh waters to protect themselves from predators, particularly the many coyotes who roamed nearby but who would not come after them through the water.

As I drove into the refuge, I imagined the tall cranes and the snow geese out in the dark marsh waters in front of me. The vast marsh in the distance felt black to me. The whole area was darker by far than the state highway had been. I had noted the day before, when planning my trip, that after passing the entry booth to the refuge, I should drive farther until I passed a narrower sandy road on my left that ran on one side of a deep irrigation ditch. I had to be careful not to turn on that first sandy road, but on the next, or I would risk driving into the ditch. But my planning had been in daylight. Now in the dark, I could not see well enough to discern one sandy road from another. I became afraid. My hands started to sweat. I wanted to cry. I had not been prepared for this more extreme darkness as soon as I got into the refuge. There was no asphalt here to reflect my car's headlights, no white lines showed me the edges of the road. I felt surrounded by a very soft darkness; it felt absorptive.

Finally I saw a sign that said "wrong way" and I knew that was my turn. While in the daytime, traffic looped the marsh in one direction only, the very early morning was not a time for traffic. I turned left onto the second sand road and began to drive more quickly. I did not want someone to come out and send me back for going the wrong way. As I drove, my headlights hardly seemed to light up the road. I turned on my brights, but they made only a small difference. The road I was driving on would take me around to the front edge of a large central area of the marsh. The dark marsh lay to my right, the irrigation ditch and a small pond to my left, backed by woods or "bosque," woods by a river. As I drove, I watched carefully for the edges of the sandy road I was on, but I could not see them. I feared driving off the road and into the marsh or the ditch.

I soon felt I was going a long way, too far for my destination—a spot next to the marsh from which I would have a most splendid view of low-lying brown mountains in the far distance behind which the first light of day would appear. Between me and that far horizon lay the marsh basin. I was worried, had I missed my spot? The darkness frightened me. Then I saw the domed shape of a metal out-house reflecting the light of my car headlights, and beyond it the vague suggestion of a sandy turnoff, a path dipping down on my left to a small parking area.

I turned. My car shook and lurched down. I had missed the sandy path and was driving through brambles. I backed my car up, pulled it forward, then juggled it, trying to position it so that my front windshield would face the marsh at exactly the right angle. Then later I could sit in my car, taking advantage of the warmth, and look out at the night sky and the early morning light show over the refuge. I turned off my headlights now. I did not want to shine them into the marsh, startling the birds. Already, half a dozen ducks had been startled and flown up.

No one else was around. I was in luck. I had wanted to be at my spot before anyone else got here. The geese out in the center of the dark marsh were making a fuss and a racket. I had heard them as soon as I drove into the refuge—the distant clamoring, clacking, throaty calling noises of the snow geese, combined with that unreflective darkness. Now I opened my car door to get out and see more exactly where I was, with my eyes not divided from the world by a windowpane. I wanted to walk around, check the position of my car.

I stepped out and almost fell down into a mess of brambles. The ground was farther below the car than I had thought. I had parked on a slope. Frightened again, I wondered where I was in relation to the road, the marsh. Outside things seemed black and cold. I stumbled through the brush and tumbleweeds, the brambles scratching my legs. As I walked forward, I found I was farther from the road than I expected. I had not taken a flashlight. I went back to my car to get one, upset that I saw so poorly without a light.

LIGHT

Now I pointed my flashlight in front of me and walked in the direction of a narrow wooden deck that stretched out over a small portion of the marsh. As I stepped onto the deck, my feet cracked a thin layer of ice on the surface of the wooden planks. The air coming up from the water below chilled my feet through my boots. I heard the quiet sound of ducks gliding by in the water in front of me, the deep gutteral noises of cranes farther out in the marsh, these birds, like me, waiting for the dawn.

I was here to see that early morning drama when the birds fly up out of the marsh and over to the nearby fields to eat. The sky would become a busy place and the light in the sky would change. After looking down into the black water below the deck, I went back to my car and stood outside it in the dark, listening. The snow geese far out in the marsh continued their muted, squawky commotion. In the woods behind me, all seemed quiet, but then I heard the low moaning sounds of birds. I looked up and the sky above me was black, except for stars and a thin white sliver of a moon. I looked into the distance to see if there was yet a sign of light on the eastern horizon. There was none. I felt happy. I had gotten here in time. I was in a complete but temporary darkness, soaking up the remaining moments of the night.

I took out my camera to try to take a picture of the black sky with the stars and sliver moon, but it never came out. I got back in my car and sat for a few minutes with the engine and heater on, getting warm, before I got out again nervously. I did not want to miss anything. I did not want the light in the sky to change without my knowing.

Outside, I was reassured to find the sky still black. I heard a wail in the woods and distant fields behind me, a long, thin cry of a coyote, then the deep hoot of a mourning dove in the woods closer by. I heard a second coyote cry, sounding almost human, and the light changed. The sky in the distance became a tad brighter. Perhaps the coyotes and birds knew the light was coming before I did, or perhaps they mourned the passing of the night. Soon a thin band of faint light seemed to hang at the far horizon, defining beneath it the undulating top ridge of the low-lying distant mountains and the flatter mesas.

The sky seemed divided in two. Directly above me, it was pitch black with the stars and sliver moon, but the sky across from me out over the marsh was an ever-lightening blue-black. In a way, the best time had passed. The sky now seemed too light to me. Yet I thought that were a stranger to arrive at just that moment, she would feel we were still in the darkness of night.

For what seemed a long time, I watched in the darkness, standing by my car, getting in to get warm, getting out to walk around. I walked to the end of the wooden deck where a crossdeck stretched horizontally to form a T out over the water. I lifted my binoculars to my eyes, hoping to see the long-legged sandhill cranes that I knew were out there in the marsh, but there was not yet enough light for me to see them. Down in front of me, the water remained black. Still, the sky overhead seemed to be changing quickly and imperceptibly, becoming lighter.

The shapes of the marsh were beginning to appear. I walked back to the land and looked out at the marsh. In front of me lay an expanse of water broken by the dark silhouettes of rushes, trees, and brush, the trees and brush sitting on spits of land jutting out into the middle of the marsh. The rounded shape of the marsh basin began to be visible, and in the distance behind it, the curved dome of a low-lying far mountain. Behind me, the trees in the woods on the other side of the irrigation ditch were beginning to take form, and behind them the huge triangle-shaped Chupadera mountain. I could suddenly see the sandy road at my feet; it was a light gray color. I could see the way my car was parked. Another car had arrived and parked a distance from me. I felt time had speeded up. Things were changing too fast. A world was appearing too quickly out of the darkness.

COLORS

I went back out onto the observation deck, where I could see the frost on the wooden planks and on the railings. I could see the wood of the deck without my flashlight now, which was a relief to me, this sudden return of vision. A silver light now touched the dark water in front of me, gleaming off it. Ducks glided among the silvery blue-black reflections of the sky. Soon, a rising white fog of early morning appeared in the marsh. Amidst the fog, the long-legged cranes stretched their elegant necks as they moved about. There were per- haps a hundred cranes in this small portion of the marsh, standing and walking among the watery grasses, some with their heads down eating; others were lining up next to each other, or landing in place, announcing themselves with a flap of broad gray wings, calling out to each other with deep resonant nasal cries, garoo-a-a-a.

This was a black and white time in the marsh. The cranes were gray, tinged with silvery white. I could see them with my binoculars now; there was suddenly enough light. Farther out behind the cranes were snow geese, visible to me as small white patches in the marsh darkness, or as a white fluttering mass. The snow geese gathered in groups of hundreds here and there on hidden ponds. Both the cranes and geese looked small and far away to me. I have noticed that wild birds have a habit of standing just beyond clear vision—or my good clear vision. Perhaps it was my eyes that made them seem just beyond clear sight. Still, with my binoculars, I could make out the shapes of the birds' bodies and their activities.

The black and white light was changing now so that tans and browns began to appear. Tan tones glinted off the backs of the cranes and off their plumed rear gray feathers. Tan touched the rushes and brown glowed up through the dark marsh waters. The surface of the water in front of me was now silvery brown in some places, silvery ink-blue in others. Everywhere, the water in the marsh was becom- ing more mirrorlike, reflecting the ever-lightening sky. It seemed to me just moments before that I had looked at the sky, but it was actu- ally a quarter of an hour ago. I looked up and several stars were still visible, but they were faint and the sliver moon looked faded. The sky out over the marsh toward the eastern horizon was lighter now, blushing blue against the old darkness. I looked down at the water to see how the light was changing on it, then up, at the sky.

I looked back toward the land, then I ran back to it. The large cottonwood trees the other side of the irrigation ditch had turned a dark yellow, a deep glowing gold. The road at my feet suddenly looked light tan; yellow tones had entered the gray. I turned around toward the marsh to see the wood of the observation deck glowing a deep yellow-brown. I felt in a race for time to take it all in. The marsh waters were now streaked with dark golden light, the tall reeds had turned a golden tan; there were reds far out, the suggestion of green. There was dark green in the water. There was suddenly color. Where at first there had been darkness, then dark shapes and gray and silver, now there was tan and color and this bath of deep gold; the golden light was especially striking on the yellow-leaved cottonwood trees. This first gold was my favorite color time at the marsh. Then as quickly as it had come, the dark golden moment was over. The trees in the cottonwood grove turned a lighter yellow, bathed by a thinner wash of color. Still, the sun had not yet come up.

The air around me felt suddenly cold. I returned to my car, stood beside it, took out my thermos, drank some coffee, and ate some coffee cake. I liked the warmth and the sweetness. Then I walked back onto the observation deck. My fingers were quickly numb from the cold when I took them out of my pockets to focus my binoculars. I looked out into the water in the marsh, which was now dark green mixed with brown. Silver-white tones shimmered glasslike across the surface. The shapes of clouds in the sky soon began to be reflected on the water's dark surface. Then the clouds and the water began to turn rose.

I looked up. Suddenly the sky in the distance was tinged with pink. A band of pink light hung above the farm fields in the north on my left. The scattered clouds in that area had pink bottom edges. The pink color soon began moving out over the farther fields, toward the river, and above the distant mesas and mountains so that pinks now marked the entire eastern sweep of the sky. I looked down into the marsh waters and when I next looked up, the curved dome of the low-lying far mountain burst into a bright glowing rose, as if lit up with a soft pink inner light. I looked away for a moment, and the rose color faded. The mountain became a light pinkish brown, though the rose color was still in the sky and on the clouds.

The color kept moving, north to south, left to right, finally hitting the large peak of a southern mountain and hanging above it. The rose colors in the sky were becoming darker now than the earlier subtle pinks had been. I turned west and the massive triangular mountain behind the refuge was a deep pink-toned golden brown. Entire clouds floating by on all sides were dark rose. In front of me in the marsh, reflections of the dark pink clouds moved across the silvery blue and tan surface of the water, making deep rose patterns shine. I was surrounded above and below by pink light. The dawn had come, resplendent with rosy glow, and it was momentary. Above me lingered two faint stars and the hazy sliver of a moon. The sky overhead was still a darker blue than the sky out over the marsh toward the horizon where the sun would come up. The sky there was silvery. The rose colors had completely gone now. Above the marsh, the sky increasingly looked like white slate. I suddenly missed the deep rose colors and the night.

BIRDS

By now more cars had arrived and were parked near the observation deck. They seemed to come with the light. I looked at my watch. I wanted to gauge how far I was from sunrise, because moments before the sun would appear above the far mountains, the snow geese would fly up en masse, by the thousands, and circle and swarm noisily high in the sky. Many of the cranes would fly up with them, then head out to the fields to eat.

I stood out on the observation deck scanning the sky through my binoculars, looking for the birds. It was never clear where the masses of snow geese would come from, or at exactly what moment they would rise. I heard sounds of geese out in the middle of the marsh. Groups of white birds were flying up periodically from the hidden ponds, then settling back down, as if practicing for takeoff.

But I was looking out into the farther distance for the larger flocks of geese that might rise at any moment, perhaps from down near the river. I did not want to miss the sudden rising of these big white birds, which I feared might be almost invisible to me. The snow geese, although large, at a distance would look like small black specks against the gray sky. There was more light now than there had been earlier, but I knew that my vision made things look darker than usual; it was as if I was looking through a cloudy lens. Objects at a distance would become small and blend in with the background. I was worried that when the snow geese rose, they would be such tiny specks that I would not be able to see them. I hoped I would hear them.

Finally I heard distant noises, but I saw nothing. I was ready to cry. I had been waiting a long time. The sun would soon be up. I regretted that Hannah was not with me. When she had been here yesterday, she had pointed out to me the distant figures in the sky when the snow geese first started to rise so that I could focus my binoculars on them.

Another woman was out on the observation deck now. She was standing on the opposite end of the crossdeck from me. I had been ignoring her, wanting to feel I was alone, but finally I walked up to her and asked, had she seen the snow geese? "No," she replied, "they're late." I felt relieved. I thought I had missed them.

That I might have missed this massive rising of white birds frightened me. I was distressed that something could occur that was so obvious to everyone, so large and present in the sky, but I would not know it was there. A sense of missing things was very much with me on this, my first pre-dawn visit to the marsh alone. When Hannah had been with me, I did not feel as uneasy. But I had wanted to go by myself this time and be alone in nature and not need anyone's help. The woman beside me and I both scanned the sky, feeling the birds had missed an appointment.

"There they go," she said suddenly. I looked up toward a spot in the gray-white sky behind a line of far away trees. Swarms of noisy snow geese looking like huge flocks of black specks rose and merged and circled and circled, then came closer, weaving, swaying, creating a moving tapestry of patterns in the silvery air. They picked up additional troops from the marshes as they moved along, circling over the marsh, then overhead, the whites of their wings visible as they came closer; then they headed out to the fields. I lifted my camera to take a picture of these frantic birds, but no picture could capture that action, the flowing movement, the significance of the dots in the sky, the light glinting off the birds' white wings and bodies. I was so relieved I could see them.

Small groups of cranes flew up out of the marsh next. The drama of the refuge was becoming slower, and more visible to me. The water in front of me was now a deep blue-gray with the suggestion of clouds in it. The long-legged cranes seemed amazingly close, standing out in the silvery brown marsh grasses. They were taking off, flapping their broad wings, rising into the air, their feathers tinted tan in the new light. They often flew in families of two and three. Sometimes several of the graceful cranes flew directly over my head en route to the fields. I could look up and see them without my binoculars now, their legs stretched out straight behind them, their long necks stretched straight ahead, their heads with that red stripe, their wings flapping in undulating rhythms of golden gray touched with silver-white. These sandhill cranes were four feet long when flying, their wingspan six to seven feet broad. I watched each crane and group that flew near me as if I had never seen a sandhill crane before.

The woman I had met on the observation deck wanted to take a picture of the cranes flying by but she had run out of film. I gave her my camera and promised to send her the photos later. She, like I, was intent on capturing the visual imagery around her no matter how small, as if her pictures would, in fact, capture her experiences. "If I lived here, I'd come here all the time," she said. "It's accessible wildlife." I liked her expression. Yet I was beginning to feel my time for capturing experience with my vision would be limited. I knew these huge cranes would be only small specks on my film and increasingly small images in my eyes in future years. So that morning, I sought to capture the colors, the dramatic changes of light over the refuge, the forms of the mountains, trees, clouds, and marsh.

The air above my head now filled with a new flock of noisy snow geese circling madly. A mass of perhaps two hundred who had not yet left for the fields were on their way. Among them, several elegant cranes flew with their legs outstretched against the chalky gray sky. Suddenly, a bright light bleached the sky and the marsh of all color, turning it black and white. The sky turned white. I looked out over the marsh toward the eastern horizon and the distant domed mountain. I had to look down and away. The new light was blinding. The sun rose. It rose too quickly, and as if without warning. First a top of a yellow sphere appeared, then that intense flash of white light. I was suddenly in a harsh world. My day felt over.

VISION

I walked slowly back to the road, near where I had parked my car, and I paced, looking down at the ground, thinking about what to do next. When I looked up, the marsh all around me, suddenly thrust into day, had turned a wheaten color. I noticed that a man was standing not far away from me, looking out at the water. As I approached him, he pointed out a bald eagle perched in a dead tree straight ahead in the marsh. He could see it with his bare eyes. It was sitting on a high limb out over the water eating a fish. I could not see the slender tree with my bare eyes. I had to use my binoculars to find it. Even then, I had to strain to see the tree, the eagle, and the fish. Struck by how poor my vision was, I felt ready to cry. Still, I could see more than I had expected.

The man left. I stood on the shore watching the marsh in the new yellowing wheaten light. A marsh hawk flew over the tall tan reeds in front of me, scouting the waters; a swarm of blackbirds flew by. The marsh was turning from tan to a deeper light gold. All the people who had come for the early morning "fly out" of the cranes and geese had, by now, driven off. I stayed, glad to be alone, and watched as the cottonwoods in the grove behind me turned bright yellow. The mountain behind them turned gold. I watched as killdeer walked on the sandy road to my side; these small brown-and-white striped birds fake woundedness to distract attackers from their nests. A group of waddling Canada geese with black necks and brown bellies crossed the road not far from me to reach the grass near the irrigation ditch, then sat as if squatting, eating the grass in the sun.

Out in the quiet yellow marsh, scattered cranes who had remained behind now started taking off, flying up with broad flaps of what looked like gold feathery wings. They glided into the air, tucking their wings, their red-streaked heads and pale necks reflecting the new golden light. I raised my binoculars and again followed with joy every crane that flew by. I was so intent on watching them that I forgot, for the moment, that I could not see well. True, when I tried to focus my binoculars on a bird's neck, I would notice that the straight line of its neck curved oddly and seemed broken in places, a distortion caused by my eyesight. But then I would focus on the larger form of the bird.

A few of the golden cranes flew to a spot on the road surprisingly near me and began walking toward the yellow cottonwood trees. I walked toward them and picked up my camera to take a picture. Although the birds would turn out small, I wanted a reminder. This place was so alive to me with its changing colors and movements, and the presence of the big birds. I was beginning to get used to the new colors, which were far brighter than the darker, pre-sunrise gold had been. This second golden yellow light began to feel special to me.

All around me was light now. I could see quite well. Still, I had leftover feelings of fear from my earlier morning hours in the dark when my vision had been more limited. The tensions I had felt when driving my car in the dark had never really left me. Although I was now looking around at a bright yellow marsh, I still saw myself driving in blackness to get here. I'd had to focus with great effort to stay on the black asphalt road and then on the sand road in the refuge in order to reach my favorite spot. I began sweating thinking of my earlier experiences in the dark, then I pushed those memories away.

This was my time to wander. For an hour in the soft golden light, I took a walk through a rear portion of the refuge, driving first to the other side of the marsh basin. As I stood deep in the refuge between the wetlands and the woods leading toward the river, I looked back at the area where I had stood in the early dawn. Surrounded by the yellow colors of trees, fields, and brush, I began to walk with the sun behind me.

As I walked, I looked at the woods by my side. The outlines of the golden and orange trees looked blurry to me, which disturbed me, but it also lent a softness. I felt bathed in the softness, the light sand color of the road, the ochre fields. Above me, the sky was now bright blue. In front of me in the marshes lay many glasslike blue ponds which, though shallow, looked deep. I walked past a pond in a far back corner of the refuge that was full of dead gray and white bare trees on which black cormorants sat on high branches like solemn Christmas tree ornaments.

At one point, a green-headed pheasant flew up noisily out of the woods at my side as I walked past. Large orange-bellied, striped-tailed marsh hawks circled over golden fields near me beside tall trees. I watched as a great blue heron stood by an irrigation ditch eating a fish. Moments later, as I turned a corner, a large cloud of white snow geese appeared and circled high in the sky, then funneled down and landed on a shimmering blue pond, turning it half white. The geese were returning from the fields. On the far side of the pond, I saw a tall white egret standing and I saw many ducks and brown and black Canada geese. The sky was clear, the feeling peaceful; the marsh seemed all mine. I walked, wanting to take in the place where I was and to stretch and be alone, and as if my movement would keep my worries away. Groups of graceful cranes, their long necks bent down, munched on watery vegetation in marshy fields as I passed, their bodies gleaming silvery gray.

I was glad I could see as well as I could. I could see well enough to take pictures. Still, I was bothered that the trees looked blurry and that try as I could to get a bird's body outlines to look clear, I could not. These were reminders that I was losing my eyesight. And yet I could see.

The memory of that November morning when I went birdwatching before sunrise stays with me vividly, with its many colors and shapes. My experience of starting out in the dark and then moving into the light has come to stand for my struggles with loss of vision and for my desires to be on my own and capable and still see. I began by driving in the dark, trying to do what I had always done before with sight. I was afraid both because I could not see well and because I was doing what perhaps I should not do alone. I needed to tell someone how scared I had been earlier when driving and how saddened by the broken outlines of the bodies of the birds. I wondered what would happen if I lost my color vision, which now provided me with such joy. I thought about that moment when the sun had seemed too bright and seemed to wipe out the night too quickly, and then to banish the dawn, the silver, gold, and rose colors. The bright light of the sun seemed to wipe out my fears, or my grounds for fear.

The sunlight, now so bright all around me, stood in my mind for vision through eyesight. With total darkness, there is no vision; with some light, there is a kind of beautiful black and white vision; with more light comes color. I wanted to feel that vision through eyesight with all its specificity and exciting color was too harsh, that the darkness was better, as was the dawn, the inbetween period, the subtle light. But I had been very afraid in the dark. I feared losing my eyesight and plunging into darkness permanently—the darkness of losing my way, of no one knowing where I am, of missing out, of facing an unfathomable blackness.

Yet I knew that when I was in the dark of the very early morning and felt afraid, I had also felt special, alone, alive in a reality no one else could see. I feared that when it got brighter, I would lose my special world; other people would come, which they did. I wanted to prefer the dark, the loss of vision. I had liked the protectedness of the dark before the demands of the world. But perhaps I am trying to make my loss of eyesight seem better to myself than it is, for I also liked what I saw later—the shapes, the colors, the movement.

I am caught, I suppose, in an invisible reality—neither totally dark nor quite light enough, a wanderer in a strange land in which I must constantly think about something as taken for granted as what I see. I must watch my step all the time, especially when in low light or unfamiliar places. I must gauge my movements to take into account the difference between the world as it is, or as it used to be for me, and the world I see. I must expect not to see.

These are difficult adjustments, even for someone like me, who takes pride in not needing the normal or the conventional supports at all times. I, who have long lived taking great nourishment from visual images, in fact thriving off a certain feeding from my eyes, must learn to lose, not to see what I might. Yet somehow I do not feel I am experiencing a loss as much as I am involved in a struggle with the negativity that surrounds me concerning loss of sight—the metaphors of darkness as bad (as loss, blindness, incapacity, disability, lack), and of light as good (as vision, clarity, truth, beauty, revelation). I am constantly trying to turn the negatives to a positive. In the marsh, I needed to enjoy what I could see—the golden colors, the shapes. I needed not to lose. Magically, I found I could see beauty no matter what the light.

I looked around now at the golden marsh and the blue sky. I was tired from my early morning adventures, so I finally got in my car and drove out of the refuge. At the entryway, I turned onto what now looked like a plain gray, cracked and aged asphalt road. The yellow dotted line down the center of the road was hardly visible; the white lines on the edges looked faded and did not particularly stand out. No rabbity blur jumped off the gray roadbed in front of me. I saw green fields with cows grazing and I did not have to strain to see landmarks. Landmarks, the concept is so visual; yet I must remember that the experiences by which I find my way are not visual. They are emotional and sentimental.

I was on my way home, back to my shared reality with Hannah, who certainly should be up by now. It was four hours since I had left. I would tell Hannah about my fears in the dark and in the very early morning before sunrise and about the rose colors in the sky. I would tell her about the coyotes howling and the birds wailing just before the first light, and that I had thought I had missed the fly out, the massive rising of the snow geese, but I had not.

TEN

Blindspots

In this chapter I explore the experience of being hit by a car that I did not see coming because of blindspots in my vision. In reflecting on the accident, I had to confront my denial of the difference that becoming increasingly blind was making in my life. Beginning with an account of the accident, this story broadens to consider issues of blindness and sight, injury and healing, and the possibility of seeing internally what no longer appears outside.

A FEW MONTHS AGO, I was hit by a car. I was walking a block away from my home and about to cross the street when a red car hit me. I was tossed up on the hood of the car, spun around, brushed against the front windshield, and thrown onto the sidewalk. I was hurt on my right leg and arm but nothing was broken, nothing severely damaged. I remember seeing the car come toward me suddenly. It was the brightest red I ever saw. I could not believe it was going to hit me. In that moment, as I flew through the air, I kept swearing at the driver, "Damn you! How could you do this to me!"

Because I swore at him at the time, I don't feel angry anymore. Though perhaps it's because my dominant feeling is disbelief. I don't really believe I was hit by that car. I don't really believe I could be hurt. I don't believe that I can't see, or can't see very well.

When the red car hit me, I was in a crosswalk marked with white lines. I had just taken three steps off the curb. It was a rainy day. The driver—whom I later saw to be a kindly looking middle-aged man with a round belly and a short white beard—was cutting the corner closely and quickly, taking a turn from the opposite side of the street. He did not see me as I began to cross. He was clearly in the wrong. But I also did not see him. I did not see a car in the wrong place out of the corner of my eye. My peripheral vision is impaired, so I have blindspots on the edges of what I see and the car was probably in one of them. I have thought, since the accident, that blind people should be able to cross the street without having someone hit them, so I should have been able to cross. But I do not see myself as blind. I see myself as a person who should have been able to see.

I take many messages from the accident. I noticed that soon afterward, I kept trying to figure out how much money I could collect from the driver's insurance company, as if getting lots of money would make me feel safe. I would not have to worry about not having money, or about feeling worthless—which is a theme for me generally, but being hit by a car probably made me feel more dispensable. So I came home and focused on getting rich. It took me a while to begin to focus on my injuries and on the physical therapy I would need, as if there, too, I wanted to deny that something was wrong with me.

I do not see well. It takes me a long time to do things I may once have done more quickly, or with less thought. I am often close to tears when I bump into things and hurt myself, or trip, or get splinters in my fingers that I cannot see. Recently, I have had to spend much time trying to get a new computer made, with large print and voices that read to me. This is something I would not have to do if I saw more clearly. Soon I am not going to drive anymore, though

I know I should not have been driving for as long a time as I have. I just don't want to stop until I can't do it. I don't want to miss it. The other day, I had a ride; I was out with my lover Hannah doing errands. I asked her to stop the car, pull it over by the sidewalk, and just sit there because I did not want to go home yet. As we sat together, I burst into tears—I was glad to be out, yet sad at the same time. The mobility of the car is one I don't often have, or not as often as I used to. That's also something I don't like to think about. I don't like to think in terms of "I used to." I like to stay in the present.

In the present, I walk a lot, which is why I was walking that day I was hit by the car. When the police and paramedics came, I did not tell them I was partly blind. I did not want the driver's insurance company to decide it was my fault that I was hit. But it was on my mind—that I was walking that day rather than driving because in the misty low light of a rainy day I would not see well enough to drive safely. So I walked and was less safe. Since the accident, I have thought that it was better that I got hit by the car than that I hit someone else. Lots of people stop driving because they get in an accident and hurt someone. But this was my wake-up call. My days of driving are now clearly numbered, because I know what it feels like to be hit and I don't want to hit someone else. Sometimes I feel that it must have been worse for that driver to see me tossed up on his red hood and spun against the windshield and deposited on the sidewalk than it was for me to be hit and hurt. But that, too, is a way of denying that I hurt, that I was traumatized. This accident, of all things, should tell me that I am blind, or partly blind. Most people who are blind are partly blind.

I remember when I first started to lose my eyesight, people immediately talked to me about driving. My neighbor told me about his brother-in-law who could not drive after he lost his vision, and the implication was that this was a sad fact. My mother asked me everytime I talked with her, "Are you still driving?" rather than "How are your eyes?" I felt that driving was a measure of my loss. People seemed to equate driving with independence and with being a complete person. I decided I was not going to subscribe to that equation. Soon I would not be driving and I did not feel any less independent than before. I told myself that drivers were dependent—on roads and cars, and people giving them the right of way. Still, I had internalized much of the equation between driving, independence, and happiness. I felt that if I stopped driving, I would be less of a person.

When the paramedics were examining me in their medic van at the accident site by the side of the street, I kept thinking about my blindspots and how they had kept me from seeing the red car coming. While the two medics moved my legs, arms, and neck, asking me what hurt, I was thinking about how I had better hide from them the fact that I do not see well. Subsequently, when the police officer came and asked me what had happened, I got off my bench seat in the van and spun around to show him how I had spun after I was hit and how I had landed, and I kept thinking, "Don't detect that I am blind. Here, let me put on my glasses. Don't look at my eyes." I feared the police officer would take away my driver's license. Before he left, he handed me a small piece of paper with the driver's name, license plate number, and address on it. The paper was wet and the handwriting small and I feared I would never be able to read it.

Soon afterward, when the paramedics dropped me off at my house, I was relieved to be intact, though not so much because I was physically okay, but because no one knew about my sight. I sat at my desk and started typing a chapter where I had left off, an ice pack wrapped unsteadily around my right leg and knee. I wanted nothing to be different. I wanted not to pay very much attention to what had just happened.

When I told a friend who is totally blind about my accident, he said to me, "You have to use all your senses." Then he added, "If you don't mind my intruding, I think people with 'low vision' have it worse. They think they see. There's a lot of denial. Be safe," was the statement he left me with.

The day I was hit by the red car, I had not used all my senses. I had crossed the street without listening for approaching traffic. Had I listened, I might not have been hit. Had I seen the car, I surely would not have stepped off the curb. But then I would not be blind, or partly blind, impaired in some way that causes me not to be totally aware.

Because my vision has been gradually growing worse, last summer I took a series of lessons in the use of a blind person's white cane, a long stick with which I can probe the ground and feel objects in my path. At first, I wanted simply to buy a cane and learn to use it, but I was told I had to have a teacher. A man came out to my house. He walked with me along the streets nearby showing me how to use the cane, feel the sidewalk, go up and down steps, know if a car was parked across a driveway and then how to get around it. As I walked with him, I learned to listen. "I'm feeling things," I said to him at first. "You're hearing them," he told me. And I learned to hear the buildings as we passed them, to hear the sound of a tree deflecting the wind, to hear the changing pattern of the air when I stepped away from a building. I learned that a sudden gust of wind and some sun told me I was at a street corner. I learned that when my feet pointed up, I was headed toward the crest of an asphalt street; when they pointed down, I was headed toward the sidewalk on the other side.

I stood on a corner and my teacher told me to listen to the cars approaching in order to know whether they had stopped or kept going. I should gauge where they were by noting the position of the loudest noise in relation to the center of my forehead. He told me to listen at traffic lights for the car movement patterns, to wait until a cycle came around to my turn, then go quickly when the traffic went.

As I walked along the streets, I often walked crooked. He told me to go straight by paying attention to the buildings at my side. The space in front of a building would be quiet, it would feel rather dead. I could walk with the quiet by my side. In other places, however, there were many noises. I walked and closed my eyes and the world without vision in which I was being mobile felt very noisy and busy—full of different ways the air felt when I approached a tree or a street sign, or was about to bump into a garbage can. I heard a house on my left, then a driveway; I felt a staircase coming toward me. I heard construction noises in the distance. I felt the sun and the wind of a corner. I walked up a hill and sensed that up ahead there was something interesting going on. People were talking. Machinery was at work. I felt that the world of walking up a street and not seeing the buildings but hearing them was richer, less flat, more busy, more alive than the visual world. Then I went back to what I could see, because it was easier and I was used to it.

I learned many techniques for the proper use of a white cane from my teacher, but the real lessons for me lay in feeling I could be mobile—without a car, without a license, without seeing. I was not less good as a person for not having sight. I'd be okay. Still, somehow these lessons I took were for the blind, or for myself when I might become more blind. My teacher did not tell me what to do if I could still see, albeit imperfectly. The fact that I could see meant I could be tricked. I looked down now at a curb in front of me. It looked quite the same as the sidewalk. I wiggled my foot on it, testing it to find where the edge was. I did not want to step down improperly and turn my ankle.

I do not take my white cane with me when I walk around the streets near my home. I carry it when I travel and when I go to unfamiliar places, but I don't use it. I do not want to be singled out as blind. I don't want someone to attack me thinking I can't see them. I don't want to think about hitting them with my cane. Instead, I worry about tripping on a hose across a sidewalk or on a piece of plywood laid down from a construction site. I go suddenly blind in the low light in restaurants, where I take tiny steps, hoping I won't trip. I am cautious near the shallow stairs on the campus where I teach and I place my feet carefully whenever I sense there might be an irregularity in the ground. In shopping centers, I put my arm out in front of me when I approach what may be an invisible glass door or wall. I already walked into one once. Often I trip when I walk on the streets near my home and I catch myself before I fall. My cane would be useful to me in all these situations. But I've left it home. I don't want people to stare at me.

The day of my accident, several people got out of their cars and rushed to help me right after I was hit. One of them was a young man who later wrote a witness account for me. "Here are the broad strokes of what I saw," his account began. "It happened around 3:45 p.m. There was a light rain but visibility was good. Road traction was good. I saw you crossing Sanchez walking eastbound. The driver of the car in front of me executed a left turn. He cut diagonally across the intersection and was going maybe 15–20 mph. You were several feet into the intersection when he hit you. You went over the hood of his car and landed on the sidewalk. He stopped immediately. I don't know how he didn't see you to begin with; you were carrying an umbrella and the corner was clear. I also don't know why he turned so close; he could have missed you had he completed the turn properly. I guess he just wasn't paying attention. I was in a similar accident about thirteen years ago; I was riding a motorcycle when a car turned left into me, shattering my hip, which then had to be surgically reconstructed. You are VERY LUCKY that you didn't get seriously injured. If you need any additional information, please let me know."

When I received the police report, included was the driver's statement: "I was coming down Sanchez (northbound) and another car was coming southbound on Sanchez. I turned to my left and didn't see the pedestrian wearing blue, and I struck her. I braked before I hit her. I cut the corner close because I wanted to avoid contact with the other car coming southbound on Sanchez."

These descriptions of the accident have a chilling effect on me. The witness's statement arrived first. Before it, I had not quite believed I was hit; I did not have a visual image of what had happened. At the time of the accident, I thought I was thrown up by the red car into midair and that I had then twisted myself around, spun, and landed on the ground. I did not know I had been tossed up onto the car's hood. Only when the police officer came, after he had checked with the driver, did I find out I had not spun around on my own, but was "propelled" up onto the hood.

What struck me upon hearing that, beyond a shock that I was incorrect, was that my main sense was at least correct—I was spun around. To this day, the accident has a "spun around" feeling for me. Right after it, people told me to be sure to look in all directions when crossing a street. This was difficult for me at first because I was afraid of all cars, and because, when I tried to look in all four directions, I was spinning again. I looked to my right, then straight ahead, then to my left, then in back of me and I could not imagine how anyone could see in all these directions quickly enough to know it was safe to cross. So I just looked right, up, left, down and right again and held my breath and started walking. If there were people at a crossing with me, I tried to get them between my right leg and any oncoming traffic. If there was no one there—and to this day I do it—I put a plastic bag or a jacket I am carrying down in front of my right leg, between it and the traffic. I want no one to hit it again. I feel vulnerable there. My memories of the accident have this sense of spinning and vulnerability, of my not being able to see enough all at once, or to see what was really happening.

My right leg is still quite sore. It is bruised deeply along its length where the car hit, and it reminds me of the accident. It easily gets stiff. I notice I often rub my leg or look at it with affection. I tell it to get better. I get internally tearful about its being hurt. Sometimes I even get mad at that driver who hurt it. I notice I don't rub my eyes, though, or talk to them in a similar way. I don't take that step into sadness. I think my leg is a stand-in for my eyes, easier to see and to talk about, easier for me to feel for. I also notice that I tell people I got hit by a car, whereas I don't so easily tell them about my eyes. I tell my friends how my leg is doing. But they have to ask me before I will mention my eyes. My leg and the car accident seem bigger and more public, thus they are easier for me to talk about. But I have to remind myself they represent my vision. My leg is not really the thing that's most hurt, my eyes are.

Last weekend, I went up the street to visit two of my neighbors. I wanted to look at a tea tree in their yard, a large feathery bush over ten feet tall of a kind I was considering planting in my yard. My neighbors, two gay men, met me with much friendliness at their front door, then led me through their house to the back, where I walked carefully down their back wooden steps watching for the edges. Once in their yard, I looked up at a towering green shrub. One of my neighbors looked at it with me. "There are a few small flowers up on top," he said. I looked up. I could not see them.

"Maybe if I come back in a week," I offered, "there will be more flowers and then I'll be able to see them. What do the flowers look like?" I asked.

"They're very bright pink," he said. Then he pointed to another tea tree farther in the distance, behind the yard next door. He raised his arm and pointed his finger so that I could follow where it led. However, I could not see the tree. It blended in with the greenery of the yards in the middle of the block where there were many bushes and tall trees.

"Does it have flowers?" I asked my neighbor.

"I can't see any," he said. "It's too far away."

My other neighbor then stepped beside me. "See that space over there," he pointed toward it with his chin. I looked generally into the distance, toward greenery. "See where it looks like a tree ought to be," he said. "There was a tree there, but it fell before we moved in. The woman who lived here told us. It almost hit the house in a big storm, but then it twisted and it fell sideways. It took out two fences instead." And as he told this to me, my neighbor twisted himself around, leaned sideways, and tottered, about to fall, acting like a tree.

I looked at him and into the middle of the block at pieces of sky between distant trees and shrubbery. These small holes looked like places where a tree might have been. But I wasn't sure which space had once held the missing tree.

"It was something," my neighbor continued excitedly. "The woman who lived here ran out of the house. She thought it was going to fall on her."

I stared, still looking for the spot that might have held the tree, feeling frustrated. Then suddenly I saw it—in one of those holes. I saw it fall toward the house, then turn and take out two of the neighbor's fences. The tree I saw did not have a well-defined shape—I can't say it really had any shape—but I saw it. I must admit I also saw the pink flowers on top of the feathery tea tree in my neighbors' yard, and I saw that tree ablaze with flowers as I knew it would be in the spring. I thought about that inner vision, and about how the three of us were standing there looking off into space at a drama that none of us had actually seen. We all imagine things no longer there; we all see with inner vision.

"Describe it to me," I often ask Hannah. "Tell me what it looks like." Then she'll describe the color of flowers by the roadside that I can't see or the markings of a bird swooping by. "Can you read that article to me," I will often ask her. "Tell me what it says." I ask her this because it is often easier for her to read something brief to me than for me to take out my magnifier and focus.

I do not like to admit that I am sad about my vision. I only admit it when I have trouble that is hard to avoid, such as being hit by the car, or when I bump into something and get hurt, or trip badly, or spill a drink such as orange juice, which is hard for me to see well enough to clean up. Then I'll have a moment when I feel like crying, and then I'll recover. Often I leave my jacket places because I don't see it when we go, and we have to go back to pick it up. Once I left my jacket on a bench in a nursery, and once in a store; another time I left the dog's leash on the ground beside the car because I did not see it fall out from where it lay beside me on the seat. Hannah and I had to drive for nearly an hour on several occasions to go back and get the items I left. I have started checking for my belongings each time I leave a place, doubting the accuracy of my sight.

I am clearly not fully in my new world of lack of vision. I keep relying on sight I no longer have. I keep expecting to be able to do things as I did them before. Then I am surprised and disappointed and I feel frustrated when I can't, for instance, just get in my car and drive to the nursery, or drive down the coast as I used to. I have to learn to be patient. I don't like patience. I have to learn new habits. I already have many of them, like checking for my belongings, and feeling for curbs, or typing without looking down at the keys, because then I'll spend a lot of time struggling to see them. I have learned a habit of putting all my things in very proper places in my study, placing my pens and magnifying glass so I can reach for them without seeing them. But there are many new habits I don't have yet.

There is another side to my loss of vision, though, which does not make me sad. I take more conscious pleasure from my visual world now than I used to. The sunsets I see are prettier for me than they ever were. Colors are more beautiful, even though I know I see them less well. When I walk down the street, everything is nicer visually for me, though blurrier and harder to focus on. I don't see the dirt on the sidewalk very well anymore, which makes it easier for me to accept living in the city. I don't see small imperfections that could distress me. I see large senses of light and color and I see shapes. I have become fond of trees because they are big and their shapes stand out.

I have also become fond of succulents in my garden—thick plants with whimsical sculpted shapes. I have a small collection of them in pots and in the ground. I am enjoying them more than flowers now because the flowers are blurry for me from any distance. I do not see their edges; they fade in with other things. Whereas a succulent plant—especially if I place it where I can see it standing out against its background—is more distinct and larger. I can lift the pot to my eye and examine it, and I can feel the shape of the plant.

Next winter, if it freezes, I'll have to take in all my succulents. The extra work is going to bother me and I'll wonder why I am keeping them, but then I'll remind myself that it's because I can't see. I am changing what is beautiful around me so I can still see the beauty. I am making sure I like what I can see, and that I can still enjoy my visual abilities even as I lose them, or as they change.

I am surprised sometimes by my ability to be positive about my vision, but I like the ability. It feels necessary, like a knee-jerk denial, but also like a life force. I'll be okay. I am constantly converting the negatives in my experience to a positive, the upsetting to just a day in the life. If things take longer, I'm going to have to enjoy the process. I find, for instance, that when I type and try to speed it up, I make mistakes and must slow down. I have to enjoy the pace I have now. When I go back for my jacket, I have to enjoy the trip. I don't want to lose. I don't want to let them get me, meaning the forces of negativity—the views that assume that my vision is less good or my life is less good now. I fight these views more than any practical problem. I say to myself, "It's not bad. It's different. You can enjoy it."

Sometimes when people ask me about my eyes, I say, "I'm doing fine. My eyes are getting worse, but I'm fine." It's true.

I think about my whole life these days. I need to have a balance. The car accident certainly upset my balance. It has caused me to feel things more intensely, so that I cry more easily, often over small disappointments.

Before the accident, I had begun to feel I was in a friendlier world than when I had better eyesight. I am still struck by the fact that people are helping me more now than I am used to. Students in my classes print out their papers in large type for me. Hannah offers me her arm when we are out. And at home, when I call to her that I have lost a pill or a needle on the floor, or broken a glass, she comes quickly. She soothes my fears, which is more important than any lost item. Sometimes people fill out forms for me in a bank or a medical center. I tell them I am partly blind and it will be faster.

Because I look into people's eyes, and have eye contact with them without my knowing it, strangers in stores and on the street often greet me and say hello very warmly. They see my baseball cap and ask me how the Giants are doing, which is awkward for me. But it creates a friendliness in the atmosphere that I did not have before. I am used to being a loner. Now I have to deal with people making computers for me, and teaching me to use canes, and giving me rides. I have a background sense that I am getting help, that people care, or might try to, which is important because of all the times when they don't seem to care, or perhaps don't know how to deal with a person who is losing her vision.

The car accident makes me notice just what my vision is right now and how I am reacting to it. I have noticed that people look increasingly young to me because my vision blurs out the fine lines and subtle skin tones in their faces. I'll see a friend who is sixty with long white hair and she will look like a young girl. Hannah's face appears frozen in time, forever as it was some years ago. Everyone I meet looks about thirty-five. This troubles me because I am aware that I ought to see age. If I don't see a person's age, I'm afraid I won't know how to act toward her, how to treat her as someone her age deserves. People seem flattered when I tell them I cannot see their wrinkles and so they will always look young to me, but I am distressed because I want them to want to look their age. I want their appearance not to be deceiving. I am afraid for myself of what will happen if it is.

I am learning that when I think about the age that I don't see in a person's face, I am seeing it in my mind. But it's a switch I'm not used to—from the outer appearance to my inner sense of the reality. I am still looking so very hard for things once there.

A few weeks after my car accident, I noticed that I began looking obsessively for red cars. I was looking for the car that had hit me. I focused intently on any red car I saw, trying to make out the model. The car that hit me was a very bright red. When I first saw it coming toward me, it looked like a true red with a bit of watermelon color in it. It looked as if the sun shone down from the sky on it alone, magically lighting it up. When I next saw the car, it was parked near the paramedics' van and it clearly seemed a dark wine-colored red. I hardly believed it was the same car. I passed it as I walked over to the van. The driver had gotten out and was standing beside it, looking concerned about my well-being. I assumed then that the initial brightness of the car occurred because adrenalin had affected my vision.

Weeks later, I looked for red cars everywhere—dark ones, light ones. Even when a car was not the right model, I stared at it, trying to make it be "the car." I looked at station wagons thinking if I looked hard enough, they'd turn into sedans. I looked at gray cars and hoped that as they got closer, they would become red. I do not see colors well, so cars at a distance often look gray to me. Thus many had the possibility for becoming red when they got closer. Black cars, too, were a candidate since they often looked red to me at a distance, perhaps because black can have some red in it. When I saw an actual red car, I felt hopeful. Then I felt severely disappointed when it turned out not to be the right car.

Several times, I thought about going to the address where the driver lived and looking for the car. But then I thought he might have it in a garage and I would not be able to see it. I did not like thinking about hanging out near his house, watching. I told myself this obsession of mine was bad and useless and that it would go away. But it didn't.

Then one day as I was walking through a supermarket parking lot near my home, there it was. It was a four-door sedan, a Toyota Corolla. Not a big car, clearly wine-colored. I walked up to it and stood beside it. I checked out the license plate number to confirm it was the right car. As I approached it, I felt that I was greeting an old friend. I stood next to its right front fender, though it was the left side that hit me, but fenders are similar. I was getting reacquainted, taking some of the sting out, some of the surreal, extraterrestrial fright that I'd felt when the car hit me. I was no longer frightened of it. It was just a car.

Then I looked at my watch. I thought that the driver was probably in the supermarket shopping, and I did not want him to come out and find me there. I didn't want him to see that I was upright, that I could still walk, because maybe he'd call his insurance company and there would go all my money. So I said a last goodbye to the red car in the parking lot. I said out loud, "Goodbye car," and I walked away, deliberately limping just in case anyone saw me.

After that, I stopped looking for red cars. I think my desire to find the car that hit me was a desire to take in what had happened in a different way. The car that frightened me was bright red. The car in the parking lot was wine-colored, and I was no longer in my accident.

I see things differently now. Red cars are receding from my attention, but I am still acutely aware of my changed vision. I move around in a world of clean streets and young-looking people. My small black dog is soft to my touch and to my eyes; I don't see her individual hairs. Once, after coming back from the eye doctor with my eyes dilated, thus letting in more light, I saw the individual scraggly white hairs on my old dog and it felt too harsh. I wanted my more blurry senses. I know that although I could carry a small pair of binoculars with me when I walk, I prefer looking only with my eyes and the minimal correction of my glasses. It's a fuzzier world than the one others see, but it's the one I see most easily.

They say people who have lost their vision often do not want to get it back. I think that's true for me. I would hate to have my vision come back and then go away again. I would hate to have to unlearn what I am now making so real. I see my world. It's full of blindspots and it's constantly changing, but what isn't?

Hannah and I are closer now since my vision loss. We don't want to lose each other, so we reach out to each other more. Hannah has learned to be a sighted guide for me, so I can hold her arm when we're out and when it's dark. She leads me with subtle clues and whispers: "The staircase turns, there are seven steps. The doors are to the right. Hold onto me." A friend of hers who is blind told her, "Tell Susan if she uses her cane, she can hold your arm in public and be close and no one will know you are lesbians." That's another secrecy of mine. These things are similar.

Hannah drives us most of the time now. I am going to stop driving soon. I don't like cars right now. Even sitting in one while Hannah is driving frightens me. I grip the door handle and ask her to slow down, although she is not driving fast. If a car cuts in on my side, I am sure I am going to die.

I am still affected deeply by my car accident, by the fact that I was hit. My acupuncturist has said to me repeatedly, "Remember, you were hit by a car. A car is big. Of course, it's not better yet." It will be better one day, my leg I mean, but in a way I don't want it to be all better. I want the reminder. What happened to me was real, maiming, alerting, a part of my life. I want to remember that I can't see, and I want to know that I can trust my ingenuity, my inner strength and sight.

Because of the car accident, I now have more respect for my own vulnerability and a greater preoccupation with my safety than I did before. The image is lasting. When I was tossed up by the red car and spun around in that amazing pirouette against the windshield, in that moment when the seemingly impossible happened, I was also tossed into the light somehow—the light of a red car frighteningly aglow, and the light of recognition. I had been previously reluctant to acknowledge the extent to which I was blind and how much that changes my life. It doesn't necessarily destroy my life; in an odd way, it emphasizes my capacity for sight.

PART 4

An Intimate Memory

ELEVEN

The Lesbian-Straight Divide

Our experiences often stay with us, not encapsulated in general terms but beneath the surface as a complex of images, bits of conversation, sensations of place, details not always accessible, but sometimes seen when recalled with an inner eye. In this novella, I present an inner vision that has long held a fascination for me. It is drawn from a time over twenty years ago that feels like yesterday, so vivid are my memories of place, people, and the nature of the intimacy. Because this story is taken from autobiographical writing I did at an earlier time, it is different in tone than the preceding essays. It is more lyrical, more intense and intimate; its narrative voice is unusually candid.

In recent years when I have visited with Anna, the straight woman in this story, neither of us could speak about this important part of our past. Our silence made me begin to doubt my memory. However, when I turned to my writing from the time, I realized I could never invent such snatches of conversation and such revealing emotions. The details I had recorded told me that it happened, she loved me then, we were close, I didn't just make it up.

In drawing from my original writing, I have chosen to create a composite by piecing together small stories to form a larger whole. Though it reads like fiction, this is a true-life account. I neither censor nor reinterpret these vignettes but present them as a past drama that remains intensely real—humorous as well as heartbreaking, full of sadness along with hopefulness, a poignant and powerful memory. The relationship recalled here marked me as a person. I emerged from it with a new kind of clarity, a self-recognition born, in part, in fire, but also from a tender and treasured part of my inner life.

As I read these stories, I again wish the lesbian-straight divide did not exist, but because it does, and because it represents an important invisibility within the lesbian landscape, I wish to describe it here. I ask the reader not to judge the reality I portray but to see in it truths about relationships between women and to recognize particularly the sensitivity of female dreams, vulnerabilities, and mutual needs. Here, then, to culminate this book, as testimony to the compelling power of lost landscapes and inner visions, is one final story.

Part One

Our Needs of Each Other

I: WHAT WAS MARRIAGE?

On the day of our trip, so tied to the others, I woke to the sound of water running. Anna was drawing a bath. Thus our mornings begin. I hear the plumbing from Anna's bathroom through the wall of my bedroom and open my eyes for a glimpse of the day. I imagine Anna gently slipping into her tub. There is quiet as I doze off, then the sound of water running, the opening and closing of the bathroom door, the opening of Anna's bedroom door, and slippered footsteps down the hall to the kitchen. In moments, there will be the whistle of a tea kettle and the smell of bacon.

On this particular morning, Anna leaves the house before I am out of bed and does not come in to tell me goodbye. She assumes I am still asleep, and I have not, as is my habit, signaled with some sound, some flush of the toilet or the start of my shower, that I am awake. This system of early morning signals, like so much in our life together, was not there at first but has grown. At first, Anna would not say goodbye when she left the house in the morning. I would know by the thick slam of the front door, the metal hinge clanking on the gate outside, and the sound of her car starting down the drive, that she had left, gone, taken off for her day. I would take a quick look out my bedroom window and catch sight of her at the wheel of her car, intent on all that would be ahead. And I would imagine her day, and what it held in store, as I might think about my own.

In time, I came to ask Anna to say goodbye to me and she would, in her hurry, after she had made up her face, a step so very necessary—the acquisition of an armor for protection from the world. After she had gathered up her purse and books and her large mug of still warm tea, and sometimes before, she would come into where I lay in bed and give me a kiss. "I'm leaving," she would say, and I would see in her face the fear, the apprehensiveness so like my own. Although often I would not think that it was my fear I saw in her brow, in the cast of her eyes, my own reluctance to get on with things, to leave this nest that is our refuge, our home.

The house where I live with Anna is nestled on a hillside out on the sandy mesa north of town. It is set low to the ground, the front entrance surrounded by an earthen wall with a wooden gate leading in to a patio and the front door. The style of the house is mock-adobe, a rich muted brown. Once inside, the space feels open and inviting. The kitchen, to the right, with high wooden cabinets and counters, is a small room where much goes on. Beyond it is a dining area. Straight ahead, the living room opens out with a high white ceiling crossed by wood beams; in the center, a comfortable couch faces a white kiva fireplace. Broad picture windows look out on the distant mountain and the vast sky. The living room feels part of the surrounding desert landscape of rolling sandy hills dotted with scrub brush and yucca, occasional cactus, irrigation ditches, unpaved roads, the cottonwoods of the Rio Grande in the distance. Throughout the house, floors made of dark red Mexican tiles give a rustic yet elegant feel.

A red-tiled hallway leads from the kitchen to our two bedrooms in back. My room is on one side of the widening hallway, Anna's on the other. My room has its own bath, a small fireplace, my bed, an oak table where I spread out my writing. Across the hall, Anna's room holds her bed and small bedside table at one end, her desk, bookshelves, and unpacked boxes at the other. Her bathroom lies a few steps outside her bedroom door, on my side of the hall.

As a whole, the house feels spacious yet private and somehow still. It feels set apart, not only because it is half an hour outside of town, but because it is emotionally apart for us, a place where we alone know what goes on. When I first visited Anna here, she seemed always searching in this house for something, as if it was her home, but it did not quite fit her. The house belongs to Anna; I rent my room, but we share the space and our living.

Anna is an attractive woman in her mid-forties, with short blond hair and an alert, sensitive face. She is expressive and insightful. She often reaches out to me, speaking with her hands as if molding her words. She and I are, in some ways, a contrast. I am taller, shyer, younger by eleven years. I wear pants and plain shirts, while Anna's style is more traditionally feminine.

"When I see middle-aged women wearing makeup," Anna told me just the other day, standing before the mirror brushing her cheeks with pink, "I sometimes think they're old women trying to be young. Maybe that's what I'm doing. Maybe everybody sees. But I still have to do it." I shook my head as if to assure her that she was different. As was I. Although, of course, we are not. Our dilemmas are common. I do not wear makeup, but I have thought to try, to one day paint my face as Anna does, to feel what it is to be behind that mask, to see my eyes lined with black becoming all the more pronounced, to articulate the basic need: "I am scared, I am hiding," Anna tells the world. "I do not expect anyone will find me acceptable." Often I have said the same to her. I have told her I put on clothes as she paints her face. "I know," she laughs back. "When you walk into a room, it's the clothes that walk in. You think you look tough. Let me tell you, no matter what you wear, you don't. You can't. People see you, darling, they really do."

I have often looked into the mirror after Anna has gone, at my own face which we both now know I believe is neither mine nor there. "It's cardboard," I said to Anna once, "I don't have a face. The one I see in the mirror, it's my father's face. You don't like yours and I don't have one."

"But you do," she answered back, looking at me intently. "It is not your father's face and it's not the face of some monster child. It's yours."

She asked me later, one quiet afternoon as we sat on the floor in my bedroom talking, to imagine looking into a mirror and to see an image behind me. I assumed she expected I would see an object, but what I saw was her standing, looking over my shoulder watching. I sought not to tell her, although I finally did, for fear that my desire to keep her always with me would cause her to draw back in fear. She did not do this, however.

As she did not draw back when I said to her on the day of our trip, in a moment of similar hesitation, "We, you and I, we are crazy." I said it twice and, the second time, turned to check the expression on her face. We were already well along on our way on that drive that took us 100 miles too far, hours longer than it should have, and began before we left.

On the morning of that day, I did not get out of bed until after Anna had left the house and when I did, it was with a sense of nervousness and anticipation. I came out to the kitchen and made tea and, while the drink usually calms me, settling demons that have risen in the night, on this particular morning, the cup shook in my hand, as my body shook, and my bowel. I got off letters, went about the "business" of the day, yet there was no real business, no real urgency other than the long drive we would later take. My fear was that I would not survive it, that I could not be with Anna, could not sit next to her in a car for the hours required without causing some dreaded end. It mattered little that I had begun to learn not to run from Anna, to resist the urge I often had to leave the house whenever it seemed we would be there alone for long together. The fear persisted, that if I was present without relief, Anna would find me unappealing, no longer full of the excitement she sometimes said was my gift.

Near to noon, I took out the pair of black pants I had just bought and prepared to hem them. "You will have to wear your 'interview clothes,'" Anna had told me just a few days before and I had taken the clue: to go with her, anywhere, I should be appropriate. And so I had finally gone to the store and purchased a pair of dress pants that fit me, despite my belief that in a few months time, I would outgrow them, a belief for which Anna kidded me: "You buy pants for how you are now. If you outgrow them, you buy others. Your clothes can change."

I heard the front door open not long after I had pinned my pants and I knew that Anna was back from her class. I came out into the kitchen then, the pants turned under to mark a length, and stood before her, aware, in the midst of this display, of how I had let her become my arbiter of dress.

"You look best," she had told me weeks before, "in soft hanging things, knit weaves, clothes that are textured and gentle. You might consider women's clothes. You know, they do make them." And then she had gone shopping with me one long afternoon which, like the day of our trip, seemed to extend forever. She took piles and piles of clothes from the racks and brought them in for me to try on, as only my mother had done before. I stood, that day, in the dressing room, my breasts bare, trying on shirts and jackets to match the pants Anna continually fetched. One suit was finally the right color but when I put on the jacket, she, too, saw. "I told you," I said, looking at my reflection, "it makes me look like a man."

Since a child, I have always dressed with an eye toward what would do that, wishing, in part, to be a man, or at least to cut the figure of an adolescent boy, and always I have drawn back from the line that seems to separate men from women, to stay just this side, feeling it took great effort to emerge as a woman and suspecting I would not get away with it. Anna has told me that she too has long felt she was somehow "getting away" with that which has seemed unreal to her, although for her what seems unreal is different: her degree, for instance, and her competence in life. "I am not smart," she has said so many times. Or, "I am not smart enough."

"You are not used to thinking of yourself as smart," I have told her in reply. "You know you are maternal. You can parent, you can give love. You don't know you can also give intelligence, share the quest for knowledge and truth you have, that has you reading all these books and studying late into the night, and liking me." For it seems to Anna that I represent truth, or at least the search for it. "Prometheus," she told me early on, "that is your myth."

"Prometheus?" I asked, not then familiar with Anna's way of referring to literature and myth for an expression of her soul. "I have seen the eternal Footman hold my coat, and snicker. And, in short, I was afraid." This, from Eliot, was one of her favorites.

"Prometheus stole fire and gave it to man," she told me, teaching. "His sin was to take from the gods, to believe that man should know."

"It is not knowledge but technology he offered," I thought, seeking to dispel what she would have me believe. Though I could not for long reject her comment that I, like Prometheus, felt vultures at my breast and that I, like he, often felt I was at heart a suffering god.

In the small dressing room, quite ungodlike, sweating from the closeness that enveloped that tiny room, I asked Anna's opinion. "Too masculine, no?"

"Yes, not right for you somehow."

I looked at the irregularity of my breasts as I undressed, the right one drooping lower than the left, and vowed that, for this new outfit, I would purchase a bra. I would become more like Anna. I would dress with my womanparts acknowledged.

"The clothes you wear," she told me once, "they are men's clothes, all your clothes are men's. You dress tastefully, what you wear always looks good. Nonetheless . . . for example, those boots."

"My favorite boots?"

"They are too big."

"They are my small boots."

"Well, they look too big. They are not in keeping with you."

The day of our trip, when I came out to the kitchen to check the length of my pants, I wore my one pair of women's heeled shoes, which I have had for seven years. I turned on my heels before Anna, the length of the pants had to be just right.

"Fine," she concluded, looking at me amused.

I lifted my shirt so she might see the waist, announcing proudly that they fit.

"Yes, they fit"—her response, as if, of course, they should.

I came back out to consult with her once more before we left, after I had put on the deep-colored shirt, the turquoise necklace, and the bra I planned to wear, before returning to change my earrings, in answer to her suggestion, her question: "Do you need a pair of turquoise earrings?"

"I never change my earrings," I replied at first, in a last hold on my ability to dress. "I have worn these same gold earrings for ten years, day after day. I forget they're there. It's a matter of principle with me."

"You might not want the turquoise, but I would. That's how I dress. The earrings should match."

I changed my earrings as well and felt quite striking, quite like Anna. Finally dressed, I came out once again to where she stood in the kitchen wrapping the present we would bring: a silver Nambé plate I had picked out in her absence, spending more than I might, because she would. I came out this time to tell her of my fear. "It's as if I never knew you," I said, "as if I were a stranger about to leave for an indefinite time with an acquaintance I have just met."

She nodded, taking it in. For she too was nervous that day. Her dress, the soft woven dress that made her look so lovely, reminded me of what she must sense I should wear. It did not, she felt, fit her right. The shoulders were too loose. I followed her into her bedroom to take a closer look where, standing before a mirror, she tugged at it as this time I looked on. I had chosen that dress with her and promised we would fix it one earlier day when we had gone shopping, intending to find a suit for me and coming home with only the dress for her. For Anna buys impulsively as soon as she sees what she likes, independent of whether she has the money, while I look and consider and wait to decide.

149

Those days of our shopping were like this day of our trip, something we had not done before together. When Anna came home in
the early afternoon, I could tell she was worried about the time the
drive would take. She said this without words, with her look of confusion as I traced our route on the map. She was faintly suggesting
that the time would have to be invented from nowhere.

"You can take a book and study on the way," I said, in attempt to
speak to her fear.

"I won't study. I get carsick. We'll talk. We always talk."

And I knew that we did. But it scared me to hear it, as if, on this
particular occasion, I would be at a loss for words. We would drive
the hours in silence. We would reach the wedding reception in the
distant town, I would not have said anything, and all the while Anna
would be wishing for someone else beside her.

The wind was blowing hard when we left the house and the
card Anna had attached to the present flew off and fell to the ground
outside the front gate. I stooped to retrieve it, as I often do, finding
something Anna has lost or misplaced: a set of papers in the house,
for instance, hidden in a folder which only I can find, although it is
Anna who has mislaid it; a pot in one of the kitchen cupboards which
she searches for more and more frantically. By now, it is a kind of joke
between us: I come up with the pot, with the folder of papers, I retrieve the card, re-establishing order for the moment, feeling I have
solved the problem which lurks just the other side of Anna's efforts.
The problem for her is that she feels she is not able, not up to what
she takes on. ("I'm an 'overachiever,'" she sometimes says.) While for
me, it is that I feel too able and so my attempts, both my successes
and failures, remind me of what could happen "if only I would . . . ,"
if only I had invested more, seen more clearly, retrieved not only the
card but some hidden jewel that lay in the earth beneath.

I handed Anna the card after I found it. She laid it back on top of
the present, tucked under a ribbon, and we walked together to the
car. It was there she announced that she would drive and my face fell.
For Anna to drive meant that I would have to give up command.

The driver often listens, the passenger talks, or at least I was taught this by my mother, who believed that drivers of cars, because they must attend the road, and because one's life is quite literally in their hands, require special care. She fed my father parts of apples, sang to him, read the signs, deciphered the map, made sure that the children in back were distracted by games, said to him always at the end of a trip, "You must be tired, dear, from all that driving."

It was not only command then, but the assurance of care I gave up when I walked to the other side of the car and took my seat beside Anna, watched her turn the key and felt the wheels back down the gravel drive. Anna backs her car out of the drive and then heads forward on the dirt road that runs past the front of the house. I turn my car and head out front end first. This is telling of a difference in how we trust. Anna trusts what she cannot see, what nobody tells her will not be there: the tenderness in a heart, for instance, the desire of a child to grow. I trust more often what I am repeatedly told, and so I seek constant reassurance: "Will you love me even if I do not talk, even if this drive turns into disaster, if I sit here beside you overwhelmed with discomfort in the fit of my new clothes?"

These were my internal questions, but right then I did not ask. I was so self-conscious at the start of that drive that, for the first two hours at least, I for once failed to see the point in talk. I felt I most certainly would not live up to some myth Anna had of me, that I was the articulate one, the one who says what another cannot put into words.

If Anna, for her part, felt a similar fear, I do not know. For she speaks less about, than from, whatever goes on inside of her. We drove for what seemed to me like days before the highway opened out south of town and we talked I do not remember of what, although most likely Anna attempted to answer some of those questions I am always putting to her: "How are you feeling, what is going on inside you just now?" questions I ask often as a child, needing to know where mother is.

Anna must have told me about her degree, about the class that she had come back from earlier upset, cast into some familiar and little explored panic in which her sense that she could do what she wanted was fundamentally challenged. And I, most likely, now learning her way, that it is all right to admit that I have doubts about my abilities, must have spoken of them. I know that after leaving view of the city, we paid attention to the roadside plants, to the many small clusters of green and gold that dot the desert landscape. Such plants are important because the house we live in is also on the desert and when Anna moved into it, the land all around was sand. She brought with her some small flowering plants, a rosebush, a yucca, and a tiny fir tree and these, for a long time, stood alone in front as reminders of another place, her mother's garden from which she had dug them up.

Since then we have made forays into fields about and claimed what grows wild: weeds and grasses, plants Anna calls "yellow plants," or "red ones," or "blues," in order to have them near the house. Drives through the country are occasions to look with longing and, for Anna, with an eye toward possession. In this way, she will make the new house hers, no longer an extension of Mama's. And I, looking with her, desire to help and am sometimes reminded of one particular plant, the rosebush from Anna's mother's garden which stands now in the walled patio outside the front door.

One afternoon, Anna called me from work to tell me that she was confused and down and I stepped outside after I had hung up and saw a full bud on the rosebush. I hesitated and then called her back. "The rosebush is blooming in the rain," I said. "There is one bud. Think of it alive and beautiful. Think of it in your feeling bad." I hung up quickly, embarrassed at my message, unsure of what to make of her silence. The next day she clipped the budding rose, brought it into the house and gave it to me. It stood in a vase in my room for weeks, never becoming fully open and bearing, I thought, some important meaning I did not exactly understand.

As we continued driving south, I felt withdrawn. It may have been my clothes. I felt hidden and uncomfortable. Though more likely it was the fear, my fear of failing, of not being able to pull it off, which was somehow tied to those clothes.

Anna and I spoke of restaurants after a while; this was a way of sharing how we had each been raised and a way, I felt then, of retreating from the present: the bare land outside, the length of the drive, the sense that it might go on forever. We spoke of expensive restaurants and how Anna had taken her children to them when they were young in order to teach them manners. I had gone to such places rarely, feeling I did not belong, resenting the rich. We were different on that score. Anna was raised to admire wealth, I with an eye toward revolution.

As we drove farther and farther south, the land spread out, distant mountains on each side, and I felt an unspoken tension between us. At one point after about two hours, we pulled off the highway to make a rest stop. In silence, we got out of the car and went quickly to adjoining stalls inside a remote gas station, each of us relieving herself spontaneously and fully. Anna bought at that station, in quart and gallon sizes, a drink called cherry cider, a treat from her childhood.

As we drove off, I thought about the rest stop, how intimate we had been, how familiar with each other, yet how much distance I felt there still was between us.

It was not until the third hour of the trip that I knew for sure we had passed the turn we should have taken east. About half an hour beyond that turn, Anna asked if I would look on the map. She pulled the car off the road and looked over my shoulder as I held it out. We stared at a spot on the map where we imagined we were and decided to keep on going, to head farther south on the main highway than we had planned, then swing east and north to reach the small town up in the mountains which was our destination.

Had we taken the proper exit, we would have approached the town more directly and would have driven an hour and a half less. But the time just then did not seem to matter. We needed to keep on going.

I was driving now and I drove quickly, the car verging on 85 miles per hour, the wheels spinning as if on their own, threatening to lurch out of control. I finally slowed down, squinted my eyes, and looked over at Anna. "I think we are crazy," I said to her. She nodded and her agreement reassured me. I was feeling very lost, lost nowhere with the day getting dark, the scrub to both sides of the road even thinner.

"We are crazy," I said to Anna again and she looked at me hard this time, as if she, too, were lost in a recognition the words suggested. I felt I was referring to an irregularity, a not quite following of the rules, to the fact of our being two women together, to our driving on, ignoring that we had missed our turn, to the partly forbidden nature of our relationship. I was also referring to the fact that we were going to this wedding reception so late in the day and at a far distance. I don't know what Anna thought. I wanted to ask her why we had kept on after we had missed our turn, but I only thought about it. I kept driving, firmly gripping the wheel.

We finally reached the southernmost point on our route, turned east from the highway and climbed up into the mountains in the dark. It was quite late when we arrived in the small town and we started to lose our way.

"Turn there," Anna said, as I jumped a curb.

"Curbs," I mumbled, "I keep running into curbs."

"You must learn to pay attention. Do you want me to drive?"

"No. I'll watch for the curbs. Just remind me every once in a while. Tell me there are curbs around."

We stopped at an all-night grocery for directions and Anna got out of the car. I watched her enter the store and felt protective of her, imagining how she would look, the expression on her face when asking or being told how to go. It would be that expression of bewilderment I knew so well, that little girl look which is often hers and which I have had to learn not to rescue. I have had to learn that Anna can stand on her own, she can cry and emerge from confusion. At home, I would often hold out an arm for her to come to me, make dinner when she was distracted, seek to convince her to sell her house, to break a relationship with a man she might marry, thinking I was protecting her when, in fact, what I sought was protection for myself, protection from the fear that if she did not do what I thought was right, I would lose my anchor, my mother, my life.

When, very intact, Anna emerged from the store, I was relieved, and she was determined to guide me: "One stop light down, then turn left, then right. There's no sign but you head on out and he says you can't miss it."

We took the turns and found the church where the reception was to be held. We passed it at first, then backed up. I pointed the car's headlights at dark letters on a sign high up on a brick wall: "Church of the Latter Day Saints," they said, which made little sense to me, though it did to Anna. Inside we stood at the back of a brightly lit room ringed by long rectangular tables around a central yellow wood floor. The room was full of very proper-looking people. We were, of course, late. I saw the bride standing off to one side wearing a white dress and veil. Next to her, the groom, our friend Daniel, had longer hair than when I had last seen him, and he stood with an air of embarrassed concern. I wanted to run up and hug him, to tell him that we had arrived, to ease my discomfort in this strange place, but Anna restrained me. It would be impolite, we should wait.

The entertainment soon began up front where a group of young women in pink and white dresses sang of purity and love; a soft-voiced guitarist played. The bride and groom stepped forward and said their thanks to the guests and to God, who surely had brought them together for some cause. A squarish woman in a white blouse and black skirt next spoke into the microphone on the verge of tears. She knew that the couple had been fated to meet, that they would serve God, that theirs was a union for all time, their love holy and good. They would bring children into the Church and carry on the Lord's work.

I did not resist my tears as they came, as I did not resist thinking of myself and Anna when love and the fatefulness of meeting was mentioned.

To my side laid out carefully on a table were pictures of the bride and groom taken just after their wedding the week before, and these I looked to with a searching eye. "What was marriage," I wanted to ask Anna, "that caused such simple joy?" What was marriage and why was it beyond us? I had been carrying the present we had brought in a box and went over to a white cloth-covered table where the gifts were piled and added ours, feeling I was giving what ought to be mine.

I did not take off my jacket, however, did not eat the clean white cake and bits of ice cream and green jello spooned from even cleaner dishes by one of the many smiling white-aproned women. Instead I stood off to one side, sipped the lemonade punch from a paper cup, and thought of the champagne I had imagined, which was, of course, not there. Mormons do not drink. Anna had told me this before we left and I needed to be told. For I was a Jew and to be among Christians, all but for Catholics, has always seemed like being among heathens to me. I told Anna of the feeling later and she did not at first understand. "I don't feel that way among Jews," she said.

"Of course not, Jews do not take the Lord's name in vain. Jews do not use the Lord's name in their every sentence. For Jews, it is not joy but suffering and triumph, it is not fate but survival that drives the Jews." But this I did not say, did not even thoroughly believe, for I was not Jew so much as alien, which perhaps was the heart of being Jewish.

When couples started to dance, Anna, who had been standing beside me, handed me her purse and went over to cut in on the groom. I watched the expression on his face as he turned toward her, his surprise: What, after all, were we doing here?, unexpected all the more because we had come so late. We stayed for half an hour, which felt like a very long time, long enough to meet the bride and the bridegroom's family. Before we left, I hugged Daniel, told him of our losing our way on the drive, how I was glad I had come and that I wished him to be happy. Yet the excitement, the real source of it for me, lay not in that wedding reception but in the fact that Anna and I had come and that we had come there together.

I was very full of the two of us that night and of my own, our own, alien quality. As if in a barely exotic dream, we left the reception in the church with polite goodbyes, intent on real food, which, by plan, we would stop for before driving the proper route back. The car was not far in the parking lot and I walked to it as if it were home. The seats were still damp with the sweat of our previous drive. I took mine beside Anna who sat determinedly at the wheel, intent on not taking any wrong turns. I laughed in relief as if it were over and our return would be easy, for now it was clear we would have a return. We were going back. We would sleep that night where we had left so much earlier in the day.

But first Anna drove back and forth on the main street in the town and I kept an eye out for some diner or cafe, some "Eat Here" that was not closed, that might offer a cloth-covered table like one in San Francisco or in the city we had left. We finally sat down at a gray formica-topped table in a restaurant that mixed Mexican with American food and had plastic flowers in vases on the tables and candles in red glass. Huge windows in front let in the darkness from outside; our table was beneath them. I sat at it nervously, ordering tea, wishing for wine. I was afraid because I was no longer sitting beside Anna protected by sideways looks and being able, when in doubt, to cast my eyes on the road. I was afraid that the food would be bad, the width of the table too much between us. Yet the tea tasted good and Anna looked at me with interest.

"Your hands," she said, as I fished a tea bag from my drink and reached for a cigarette, "I love your hands." I was embarrassed yet pleased, for I could no more hide my hands than I could the questioning smile on my face.

We stayed quite a while at that restaurant, as if it were merely next door and no drive stood before us, and we talked of our relationships with people. There was one woman Anna and I both knew, an artist. She made Anna uncomfortable. I liked her. "Maybe it's her size that discomforts you," I suggested. "That she's large. Big women, for me, they are mothers. I long to crawl in, I want to nestle in their laps." For Anna, however, it was old women who were mothers and there was something, I thought, far more safe in that.

157

We talked on and on but the point of it was that the restaurant, before we left, became a place, our place, converted from plastic flowers, formica tables, and huge dark windows to a break in the day that was close and familiar. On the way out, heady, as if the tea had been wine, I confused the money I was paying for the bill with what I wanted to leave for the tip and had to return to exchange it. Anna and I stood at the cash register, waiting for others to pay, and picked out gum for the trip home.

On the drive back I talked, and so did she, far more easily than on the drive down. We continued talking of our attractions and our needs of other people. We spoke of men and of women. Anna said she looked to women to share feelings about music, art, psychology. She looked to women for personal closeness. From men, she looked for less: for the figure of a father, for security, an ability to dance, to make the world safe. I said I looked to men for intelligence and smartness, to women for deep comfort. We drove fast in the dark night, talking of relationships with others intensely, and only lightly of the relationship between us. Yet this was there too.

After driving the hours which seemed this time to pass quickly, we left winding back roads for the highway and finally came upon the city in the north, then headed past it to the smaller town, the post office, the dirt road that leads to Anna's house. She pulled into the driveway. I opened the car door and got out. As we stood outside together next to the car, Anna pointed up at the sky. Stars appeared very clearly. She turned to me and asked their names and I wished I were an astronomer.

Inside the house in the kitchen, which now was cold but warmly lit, I poured myself a glass of scotch. Anna also took a drink and we walked down the hall with our drinks into Anna's bedroom. She took out a magazine, intent on her nightly ritual of reading something of the world before admitting sleep. I kissed her behind the ear.

"We kept going," I said to her after a while. "It is typical of us that we kept going."

"Yes," she smiled.

"Do you know why?"

"No. That kind of thing is what you like to figure out. I do it but I don't know why. Sometimes I think I don't want to."

"Do you think we are crazy?" I asked a few minutes later.

"Yes," she responded, "I think we are quite crazy."

She put down her magazine and reached for her scotch. "I am your child," I said.

"You are much more than a child to me."

Then she lay back. "It was worth it, don't you think?" I asked into her sleep. She mumbled back something not quite audible, words from a dream, another trip. And I thought of words said earlier:

"You may not want the earrings to match, but I would."

"People see you, they really do."

"You must learn to pay attention to curbs."

"Those boots, they are not in keeping with you."

"I never go to sleep easily," I once told Anna. "Sleep is always an interruption, a time out from the day that I very much fear." In the morning, I told myself this time, I would wake to the sound of water running. I would wake to Anna's kiss or to her goodbye. I would look at the sun and bury my head ever deeper under my pillow. In the morning, there would be answers. The main one, probably, would be that this day would merge with all the others. Though of course I would try to keep it apart, to learn from it some particular and much prized lesson. So that in the end I would not feel lost. We would talk of our trip and Anna would surely question my fear: my fear of her, of the changes, of the world in which we traveled, and then we would go on.

II: A FORBIDDEN SEXUALITY

I always felt there was a distance that belied the closeness between Anna and me. I had first met her when I invited her to speak in a class I was teaching at the university. Subsequently, I sought her out as a psychotherapist when I lost my job for the next year and felt rejected and alone. I soon began helping her with her dissertation and we began to be friends. I moved into Anna's house temporarily at first. Then she suggested that I stay and that we extend my psychotherapy into our living. She would help me to know my past emotional wounds and heal from them, using a re-parenting approach she specialized in.

From the beginning, I knew that Anna felt she had to be cautious with me because the world disapproved of intimacy between therapist and client. Simply living together was intimacy, and sexual intimacy, or anything leading to it, was many steps further prohibited. Additionally, I felt that the world disapproved of lesbianism, though much more implicitly, and this taboo created a line between us that was hard to cross. Repeatedly, however, we sought to cross it, reaching out to each other.

I remember a time when Anna did give in to her sexual feelings for me. She rejects that time, avoids talking about it, thinks it was a mistake. Our sexual involvement began without my knowing, a few months after I had moved in with her. Two friends of hers came to visit and we went out to dinner with them. In the restaurant, Anna and I sat across the table from her friends, John and Nancy. Several times during the conversation I put my hand to Anna's back. She did not touch me in return, or smile over at me, as I had expected she might, but rather reached for her coat on the back of her chair and pulled it around her shoulders. On the ride home as we sat in the back seat of the car, Anna said she was cold and again I put an arm around her. Again she seemed to ignore it.

She slept that night on the couch in the living room. Her friends stayed in her bed. After they were asleep, I went into the living room to talk with her, as was our habit at night, but she said she simply wanted to go to sleep.

Her friends left the next day, and that evening, Anna wanted to go to bed early and alone. The following morning, I came out to the kitchen and found her already dressed, standing at the counter going through her papers. I felt I must have done something wrong. My hand at her back had felt so unwanted, our sleeping had felt so separate. She finally looked up at me in answer to some statement of mine, some asking if I had done something to offend her. "No, you haven't," she said. "It's nothing you've done. But I must tell you. It's no good your feeling like a bad child."

"I was feeling like that."

What she said next surprised me. "Do you remember that night last week when you asked if I was in love with you? It started then. I hadn't thought I was. But when you said it, I knew. While my friends were here, I had these strong sexual feelings for you. That's why I pulled away. I need to draw back. But I wanted to tell you so you'll know. So you won't misinterpret."

"Were you afraid your friends would know?"

"That was not what I was afraid of."

For the remainder of the day, Anna seemed as if thrust in some deep depression, some inner place from which she looked out only occasionally and saw me. I did remember the night I had asked her if she was in love with me. We were standing in the kitchen looking into each other's eyes. I touched her on the shoulder. She walked away without answering.

"When do you feel it?" I asked her now.

"All the time. In many little ways. When you kiss me behind the ear, when you touch me, especially then, when I look at you. When I go into my room to get away, I can't study. I can't work. I want you."

As we sat close together on the couch that afternoon, Anna told me she was scared, scared to move, scared to touch me: "I can't. If I do, I won't stop."

"What would happen then?"

"I would tear off your clothes. I want to rape you. I have never felt like this before."

"Just hold me."

She held me gently, putting her arms around me. After a while, I turned to her. "I trust you now," I said, "more than I have ever before."

"You should not need this to feel you can trust me."

I tried to lay her back then, to relax her, kiss her. I wanted her to give in to how she felt.

"Don't. Please don't," was her reply. "It's bad. I must not."

We got up and walked over to the broad living room window that looked out on the desert. "I can't," Anna repeated. "It's not right. I need to go dancing. I need to find a man."

"Stay with it. Stay with me. Please don't take it somewhere else."

But she was deep into the inner place again.

Late that day, she drove me into town to a garage where I was to pick up my car. As she left me off, I could see the fear still in her face.

"Go to your dancing class," I said to her. "But come home. Don't go find a man."

She nodded.

That night we lay together on the couch. We fell asleep in each other's arms, drifting in and out of touching and holding. My kisses met with her no's: "Please don't. I can't." Yet there were also times that evening and in the days that followed when I stood or sat near Anna and she held me without my asking, when her fingers traced the outlines of my breasts.

The next few weeks were often mixed like that. Anna would speak to me of how she felt and I would be reassured. "At work, when you called me this afternoon," she would say, "after I hung up, I sat there pulsing. It's never been so strong. I can't work without thinking . . ."

She looked tired during those weeks, like a woman distraught. People commented at work. They asked her what was wrong.

"I am happy," she said alone to me at home. "I'm glad I have these feelings."

Often during that time when I went into the bathroom to comb my hair or change my shirt, I would look at myself in the mirror and wonder at what she saw, what was different. I would wonder about how I might act or dress to appeal to her more so that she would not pull away from me.

I told Anna of this and she was not pleased: "It's enough what you do when you are not trying, when you kiss me without thinking, like when you're saying goodbye. You don't have to seduce me. That should be a lesson to you. Don't make it into more."

Yet in many small ways, I continued to try.

Finally one evening, Anna told me she had made a decision. We were standing in the kitchen by the counter. "It's immoral," she said. "I could not live with myself. I may feel what I feel, but I will not act on these feelings. I promised you when you first came to live with me that you could be like a child to me. I want to give you a home so you can feel safe here before you move away. I want to nurture you. This would be betraying you."

I understood and I did not understand.

163

After several weeks of finding then drawing back from the line that seemed to Anna to speak of betrayal, one night as the two of us lay in her bed where, by then, we were spending the nights together, as we lay on smooth sheets in the soft light of a bedside lamp, I reached down between Anna's legs and quickly she came to orgasm. I did not know it had happened; she seemed so alone.

Two nights later, she reached down as if obliged and touched me, then drew back. "I can't," she said. "I feel sick. I am too afraid."

The next afternoon when I stopped into her office to see her, she looked upset, more distracted, more into the deep place than at any other time in all those weeks. "I've been sick to my stomach all day," she told me.

"You've been scared."

"Yes."

"I once had that fear, the first time with a woman. I think I still do."

That night we talked of women. "My mother. For me, sex is always 'bad,'" Anna began. "I had a dream last night that my mother was present and then the feeling was sexual and you walked in as a presence, a ghost. I should not. It's bad."

Later that week, Anna and I took a drive south on business. Coming home we stopped at a bar in an outlying town. As we sat at a private table having drinks and talking, Anna's eyes became tearful. "If I were a different person," she said. "Damn my tears. I can't say anything without crying. If I were different. If I were truly healthy, if I were all the things you think I should be. Someday, I might be able to live with you. It might be best for me. I think it would. But I'm not. I don't know that I'll ever be that person." She looked at me, then she looked down into her drink, then out a window to her side toward a future I knew we would not have, but I shared the dream of it at that moment.

Back home that night, we lay together on the living room couch. Anna took off her pants and hose and again came to orgasm as I touched her. We went to bed, saying nothing of it.

A few nights later, she sat up in bed soon after I began to stroke her breast. "It's not good for you," she told me. "You think that if you are very good, if you perform well. If you're skillful enough. But don't, don't do it anymore. Come to me, get what you want this way." Then she held out her arms and I came to them as a child and lifted my face to kiss her.

"I am not only a child," I said.

"I know. But be a child now, for yourself, for me."

We took a trip up into the mountains the following weekend to see the golden fall colors, and as we stood under a quaking yellow Aspen, I wanted a closeness with Anna that she seemed to push away. On the ride home, it was dark and had begun to rain, but the car inside felt protected and warm. As I drove, Anna turned to me. "With a man, I don't feel as threatened," she said. "It is as if there's a line between him and me. With a woman, the line is not there. It's more like merging with a woman. Do you feel that way?" she asked, "that it's more of a oneness, less safe?"

"I don't know. I choose women who are very different from me. Maybe that's why. Are you saying this is how you have felt with me, that the merging would be too great?"

"I think I'm saying that, yes. With two women, it's all softness. I've always felt I needed a hard body against mine."

"My body's pretty hard."

"No, not really. There are curves."

A few weeks later, over Thanksgiving, Anna went back East to be with Marc, the man she planned to marry. He had moved there for a job the spring before. While she was gone, snow fell at the house and I wished her with me. She called me several times. She was writing a paper and she wanted my advice. She said that she missed me.

Soon after she came home, we were lying in her bed one night talking when Marc called. Anna hung up the phone, putting it back slowly on her bedside table, and turned to me. "I want to explain," she began. "I didn't tell you, but Marc has lost his job out there. When I was visiting him, I told him to look into the plant where he worked here before he left. He was calling to tell me he had done that. I don't think he'll come, I really don't, but it is a possibility."

I tensed and felt myself shake inside and I may have begun to cry.

"What I am giving to you, I should be giving to him," she said. "What I want to do now is, I want to transfer my sexual feelings from you to him. I don't know if I can, but I want to do it. I'll try. I have to."

I struck out then quickly with my fist and hit her on the arm again and again. "I hate you, I hate you, I hate you," I said. "You don't have to transfer them."

Then I left her room and went to mine. Though soon afterward, I came back. "I'm sorry," I said.

"You were telling me that you loved me. I knew that."

"If Marc comes, we won't be able to sleep together anymore."

"He'll go away sometimes on business, he did before. We'll sleep together then."

In the next few days, I broke many things—a small table, a dozen bricks, my tape recorder, a necklace from a previous lover of mine. Anna stayed up with me through one long night when most of it happened. She was in turn angry with me, then helpless, then she held me as she might a much disturbed child. When I broke several dishes that we had been eating our dinners on, she became angry again. Finally she came into my room and slept with me on my bed. In the morning, her eyes, like mine, were red and we did not talk much about why.

We soon began to talk of a trip Anna planned to take to California over Christmas to see her children, all grown—a daughter and two sons. She asked me if I would go with her.

"I want you with me wherever I am," she said as we sat on the couch by the fire, her eyes becoming full as she held my hand. Moments later Marc called. She asked him if he wanted to meet her there too, and she did not at first seem to understand why I would be shaken.

As it turned out, Marc did not want to go to California, for he had been offered a job here and would move back soon after. However, he did come for a visit one weekend between Thanksgiving and Christmas after Anna called him to say she wanted to talk with him. She would fly back or he could come out here. When he came, she told him of her feelings for me, and she told him that she and I had made love. She was, I knew, desperately afraid that he would reject her, he'd not want to come back.

"He won't take it seriously," I said. "Men don't."

"You were wrong," she reported to me afterward. "He took it very seriously. But he still wants me."

"What did he say?"

"He wanted to know how it would affect my relationship with him. Did he have to be afraid I would leave him for you? I told him no. I told him I thought it would enrich it and that I wanted you to stay. I want him to love you as I do."

One night after Marc had gone, as Anna and I sat up late talking, I turned to her, "You are bringing Marc back because then you won't have to—"

"Yes." She knew before I had it said. I was reassured by the depth of her feelings, for her bringing Marc back felt like an acknowledgment of the power of our attraction.

At Christmastime, Anna and I went together to California, where she visited with her children and I visited with old friends. On my birthday, a few days after Christmas, we took a walk in the foothills and felt the new growth, the luxuriance of the trees and green that we both missed. On our walk through the woods, I felt many silences and a distance between us. That evening at dinner in a restaurant, however, Anna took out a small box and lifted from it a gold bracelet she wanted me to wear as I did a chain around my neck, always, never taking it off. The clasp on the bracelet was stiff, but we worked at it to make it fit.

The next evening when I came to say goodnight to Anna at her daughter's house, it was late and Anna's daughter and her son-in-law were asleep. Anna was sitting up alone on the couch in the living room, where she would later sleep. She was wearing a deep blue silk robe and had a drink in her hand. She stood to get me one. Then she took my hand quietly and led me to sit beside her. She held me close and kissed me. I kissed her back. She rested her head back on the couch for a moment. Then she held me to her even more tightly and cried, her large tears rolling slowly down her cheeks. "My deep river flows only for you," she said.

I said nothing and let myself be held, fearing her feelings for me would go away, that she had only spoken so passionately because she had been drinking. I also felt this was a moment to remember; I so wanted to believe her words were true.

I left that night both elated and anxious. Anna, I supposed, soon went to sleep. We flew home the next day and were alone in the house for a week before Marc came. I had asked for the time, hoping to mend what seemed to me broken or lost between us. Though, as I explained this and looked into Anna's eyes, it was clear she did not feel this same need.

"It's not broken, not lost."

"But I broke things."

"So did I."

III: "IF I COULD FIND A MAN LIKE YOU"

One of the first things Marc did when he moved back was to take out his wallet and show me a picture of his son, and then one of Anna. "That's my honey," he said, pointing to her. Then he told me that it was all right with him that I lived in the house. When he was living back East, he had been relieved because someone was here with Anna, so he worried less about her. It was all right that I stayed around a while longer. He would be with her forever.

I was hurt by his words, his sense that I was the visitor, that he could call her his honey and I could not, that I was, for him, primarily a being who took care of Anna, like a watchdog might a precious property, who filled in time until he could be with her.

"I see things in terms of roles," he told me on one of those first nights when he and Anna and I sat up late talking at the dining table trying to make things all right between us. "I see you as taking the husband role and it threatens me," he said. "Because then, who am I?"

"I'm not the husband," I started to reply. But I had to admit that I did things he understood that husbands did. I drove the garbage to the dump, looked after Anna, cleaned the floors, cared for the dogs.

"So I'm the husband," I said. "Partly I am. You've got to learn not to see it all in roles. Then you won't be threatened."

"Society recognizes marriage," he went on. "I want to marry Anna. People have ideas of a husband and wife. When we go out to dinner, that's how they treat us. A man comes with his wife. They assume certain things about the relationship. I do too. I don't know what you are. I keep trying to put you in a role and you keep saying no. Anna told me she has a relationship in which she cares for you as if you were her child. She wants to nurture you and help you have stability during this time in your life. You are the child; she is your mother. I can accept that. But now you tell me you're more than that. I don't know if I can live with it."

I looked at Marc as he spoke, at the square set of his head, his prominent brow, the way his eyes were deeply set. I watched how he walked quietly in the house, heard the stiff, formal way he spoke with Anna, and thought he would take care and be giving toward her, though I never trusted he would care for me. He was a mechanical engineer and not a subtle person.

After he moved in, the weekends became a time for him and Anna to do things together—plant in the garden, buy furniture for the house, talk of cutting holes in the ceilings for solar. The television was brought into the living room, and evenings, as a rule, were spent around it. Anna did not want to be with me out of Marc's sight in the house. She was uneasy spending time in my room. She would sit up with him in the living room watching television, her hand gently rubbing his belly, telling him in this way that she cared. I looked at them, saw his arm around her, and felt a longing. "I want someone to adore me, someone who will love me like that," I told Anna.

"You'll find someone. And I hope, for you, it will be a better match."

"I think it would be better for you and him if I were not here."
"I don't know about that." She looked content.

Anna no longer spent afternoons lying on the couch depressed, as she had before Marc came. "I haven't been settled in years," she said.

She and Marc now went as a couple to parties. She used the term "we" often, referring to the two of them. I felt confused, wanting her forever separate. With me, she had always been cautious, reluctant, fighting all but the ways in which I was like a child to her, or the ways I helped with her studies or work—the more formal, structured ways of relating between us.

After Marc came, Anna and I tried to include him in our personal talks, but he found them too heavy. We cooked meals in a large pot that would last half a week, rather than making late-at-night grilled cheese sandwiches; we bought more meat than before and there was always beer in the refrigerator. Marc wanted to eat at the dinner table, not by the fire in the living room, as we had done before he came. "We ate by the fire before, I like it too," Anna said to him, seeking to override his distrust of me.

Anna's brother, who lived in town and with whom she was close, had taken Marc aside right after he arrived and told him I was a "manipulator," that I was too powerful in Anna's life. Marc told me he did not take it to heart, though later he would use those very terms to describe me to Anna, suggesting he thought her brother was right.

Anna had such great dreams at the start. "I have this fantasy," she told me, "that after a while, it would be okay if Marc and I were in bed watching TV and you wanted to come in and sit with us, that Marc would welcome you as I would."

"I had the fantasy too," I told her. "But without the TV. That I would come in and you would hold me and he would too."

At one point, Anna wanted us to read Shakespeare aloud together one night a week, which we did for a while, the three of us sitting by the fire. The first play we read was Lear, and I was Cordelia. Anna knew the plot, but neither Marc nor I fully understood.

One evening as we sat by the fire talking after reading a play, Anna turned to Marc. "You are my earth, my ground," she said to him. Then she turned to me, "You are my air, my excitement. Without you, I could not breathe. I am fire. I need you both."

I tried to be friends with Marc for a while, but it did not work out.

Soon I started writing stories, "The Anna Stories," I called them, about my experiences at the time. It is a quiet afternoon here out north of town, my stories began, where the land, with its sand and brush, rises and rises against the sky. I moved in last summer one rainy night when the electricity went off and the four kittens and one calico cat I had brought cried as if in some primitive pain all the long drive. The kittens I put in a large cardboard box out in the garage, and I, soaked through, sat in the dark and talked as a child come home.

We sat side by side, Anna and I, on that couch placed precisely wrong for the view. We sat in the dark by the light of candles, each of them having seen most of its use. We sat lit by half a dozen glowing stubs, awkwardly, it might appear. My clothes were wet through from the rain, yet I declined an offer of dry pants and shirt, because I was not feeling cold, because I was finally where I belonged. I had been in the house only three times before and each time, Anna had held me, held me for hours as a tiny one, a little girl with a teddybear and overalls and unruly curly hair.

I did not know then that I would move in, that one of the back bedrooms would become mine. I hide there. I retreat to write. Anna now sits studying. I have played her a record that she will only partly understand—of one woman singing to another. "You still want the connection," she says. This much she grasps.

"Tell me," I have asked her, time and again, "tell me that you love me." And she has responded, often enough, and I have not heard— so afraid, as the little one must have been afraid, that none of it could be true. To be a child, for me to be a child, that has been my refuge and Anna's protection.

"My deepest feelings of love have been for my children," Anna has told me more than once. And I have responded that my deepest need is to be held and loved in just that way. Yet it is the woman, not the child, who so often has put an arm out to Anna and kissed her, gently, behind the ear.

"Your gentleness," she says.

"My womanness," I answer.

"It is not because you are a woman."

This has been difficult for me. Especially now with Anna's "man" come home, a man who, too, is child to her.

"He's more immature than you. He does not feed me as you do. But I need him. I need a man," Anna has told me. "If it were not Marc, it would be someone else. If I could find a man like you . . ."

That rainy night when I moved in with Anna, I expected to stay only a few days, a time between all my other plans. Yet it has been eight months and I have not yet left. Anna said at one point, "I'll be relieved when you go. Then I won't have to deal with my feelings any longer. I will always have them inside, but I won't have to confront them directly."

The start of the year, when I thought I would leave, has long passed. My living with Anna seems a time out of time.

I have begun to wear jewelry since I came here, as Anna wears jewelry, for without it she is not dressed. Today I said to her: "I look at you and you are so lovely. I feel awkward and ugly about myself." She shook her head no and remarked on the fact that she liked that I was wearing jewelry, as if it became me, somehow completed me. Often she has told me that she finds me beautiful. Gradually, largely because of that, I have learned to look closely in the mirror. Anna came in the other morning and found me looking at my reflection. "You caught me," I said. She nodded, "Good."

I have grown thin since I have come here, this a sign of my fear. I somehow feel that if I am thin, the world will not hurt me. If I am small, I will be protected.

Tonight Anna came into my room and held me, a small taste of what it was before, when we would fall asleep in each other's arms. She came into my room and held me because she was drunk, I thought, her one night to allow that since now, as a rule, she is not drinking. When she does not drink, she is more tight, rigid in how she deals with her body, more afraid in how she touches me. But tonight, briefly, she held me close in the old way. I was wanting my mother, I had told her, wanting my real mother, whom I had spoken with earlier in the day, who was about to take off on a trip to some islands with her man friend of the moment. I told Anna that I was afraid my mother would not come back, that she would get lost in all the changes of planes and boats. I did want my mother tonight, as I suppose I have for a long time. I heard her voice in my mind, musical, it seemed to me, as mine might never be. I saw her face, soft and afraid and covered with doubts.

As I often see Anna's face. I forget my own for hers.

It is hard for me to accept that Anna will not be with me forever, that one day in the not far future, I will have to leave her. Her man, Marc, worries because he feels inferior to me. He told Anna this today. He feels I am smarter than he is. I imagined facing him and telling him, "Yes, I am. But you have something I lack. You are a man."

I told Marc one night last week that I had moments of loving him. I wanted to tell him this because so often he tells Anna or me that he does not like me; he wants me gone. I wanted to shock him with my statement of love, but also it was true. I told him how one night last week when I'd come out of my room and found him sitting by the fireplace building a fire, his cheeks all pink from his bike ride home from work, I had felt that he was tender and beautiful and I had loved him.

But that did not seem to matter a few days later, when I awoke to a fight between Anna and him, heard him telling her he simply did not like me. "Maybe it is not her," he said, "just her behavior. But anyway, I don't like her."

The days go by quickly and the nights are long. Tonight Anna and Marc sit watching television in the living room. I anticipate they will make love later on, because she is drunk, and for the same reasons she was able to touch me, she will be able to give herself to him.

174

I imagine Anna holding Marc in bed, as if he, too, were her child, a little boy, and loving him that way. Though more often, I imagine him on top of her, penetrating, she holding onto him, surrendering, telling him how he is wonderful, how she needs him, that she loves him. I have replayed the scene many times, most nights, in fact, and by now can imagine it with cool disdain.

I go out to get my cigarettes, walk across the broad living room where Anna and Marc are watching television. "You have some cigarettes over here," Anna says, pointing to the table beside her. "Is that what you're looking for?" I nod yes, not speaking. I must speak less, I tell myself, I must convey more with my body, as Marc does. My words too often get me in trouble. Marc cannot stand me because of them, he tells Anna. I feel I am too powerful, too direct in my words, and sometimes I use too many and get lost.

I came back into my room and looked in the mirror; I found my face telling about the sadness inside. My shoulders were high—a sign of my fear, Anna has told me—and I hoped that she had noticed as I stooped to pick up my cigarettes.

I hit Marc several weeks ago, slapped him across the face when I overheard him telling Anna that I should go, that I should leave this house. I walked into the dining room where they were sitting at the table, told him he was an ass and slapped him across the face, then ran out of the house and drove away in my car, shaking. There was relief in the slap and I felt he deserved it. Yet I came back and apologized. I walked up and stood before Marc, took off my glasses, said I was sorry and suggested that he hit me back, but he did not. I remembered I had once before dared him to make me leave when he threatened he would, and, similarly, he had backed down.

At moments like this, Marc seems to me a coward, though possibly he simply overshoots with his dares. He cannot make me leave because the house is Anna's and she has said she will not ever tell me to go.

I wish I did not love her. I wish I had not raised all the hurt of the child who cannot feel loved. I wish she had never held me for those long nights, never slept with me, never come close. But really I regret none of these things. To do so would be to deny Anna's importance to me and it would deny my sense of what I need.

I found a small, black puppy at the pound several months ago and brought him home, to give us a baby, a second child, a little one who would distract me around the house. One day he got onto Anna's bed and in anger I picked him up and dropped him from on high to the floor outside the bedroom door. He was hurt and yelped and cried and I stood looking in horror at what I had done. Anna came to me then and put her arms around me. She brought me to the bed and held me as I cried. "As you love him, you will learn to love yourself," she said.

Another night, I had a terrible headache, then a stomach ache, and I could not sleep. Anna, awakened by my tears, heard me yelling out in pain. She came to my bed and lay on top of me and held me down so that I might go into the bad place—the emotional place where my feelings tunnel down in a never-ending spiral. I never got all the way there, I was too afraid. But the promise of going there stays with me still, the feeling that I must and the doubt that I ever will.

Like that was the night Anna held me as we sat on the couch and I was to her as a child. All of a sudden, with her hand at my back, I began to flinch, as if her stroking hurt me. I kept on doing this, feeling in pre-birth. The pains were in the womb, I was flinching, trying to break free and could not. I needed to be turned around and pushed. Yet I could not speak, only writhe in Anna's arms, responding to the imagined pain of her touch. She touched me at my back again and again as she held me tightly to her, so that I might feel and begin to know.

I have only begun and I worry that much of what I've dreamed may never come true. I may never go far enough into the tunnel, or turn around sufficiently to be reborn.

One night as I sat with Anna at the dining room table, back before

Marc came, she turned to me and said "I love you." I flushed and ducked, as if I had been hit.

Another night Anna cried for her own mother as she sat up watching television very late, wanting to stay up forever. Though finally she went to bed. In the morning when she woke, she was still full of tears. I held her and told her to be little, like me, and for a while, I was her mother.

I am Anna's mother often, more often than I know. I have set up my typewriter at her mother's desk, which is in my room. I went to the same college Mama did, and I, like Mama, am in Anna's eyes an "intellectual." And also a very frightened child.

In part because of her mother, Anna needs reassurances that are often quite conventional: a nice house, a husband, a moral life, a Ph.D. I need many of the same things, but for different reasons, and I was raised to have them while she was not.

Anna expresses her passion when she is drunk. I express when I write.

My puppy sleeps in his small bed outside my bedroom door. I do not know why I am here. I do not know if in the future I will look on this year as my greatest trial or my greatest gift. I feel that I learn. I know that now when I look at those I might love, I look in their faces for the child. The child in exile, the child who needs to be set free. I know only sometimes that I am that one.

Anna has come into my room tonight. She has held me and I have talked to her as I most like to talk, as the little girl with the many small things that must be said in a tiny voice before sleep.

She strokes my head and tells me she thinks in everyone is a part that is the vulnerable child. "You have a lot of that vulnerable child," she says, and I turn my chin up and give her a small kiss. I ask about the nights she is drunk, saying I get afraid because she is different then. I do not know whether to trust her.

"I'm the same inside," she says. "I'm stable that way. On the outside maybe I change. But not inside. You can trust that."

She leaves and I am quiet and not sad as I was. The affection, the ability just to talk, the little nothings between us, these are immensely reassuring for me. They work against all the other times and I need them.

"It is hard for me," I tell Anna, "because of who I am."

"It would be hard for anyone."

Because it is hard does not make it wrong, I later tell myself, since so much of what I know cautions differently. I feel often that I should run, should not be here, that the only thing that keeps me sometimes is my room, with its oak table, its rug the color of the earth outside, its white, curved yet untiled fireplace. "It is illegal to burn a fire this way," Anna has told me, "without a protected area in front." Yet I burn the fire safely.

A few days ago, when I drove away from the house, Anna and Marc were planting outside. They looked up and waved to me. I did not know what to make of the friendliness in Marc's face. "Are you real? Will you be my father? Will you be good to me?" I wanted to ask.

When Anna and Marc first left that afternoon, to look higher up on the hill for plants they could dig and bring back here, I wanted to run after them and to ask Marc to hold me. I ran out of my room to the back door but stopped short, afraid. It was not my place. I might be asking too soon. Marc might feel overwhelmed. He might hug me and grant nothing.

It was only last week, after I had knocked on Anna and Marc's bedroom door and opened it and stood there and said to Marc, "I don't like it that you don't like me, that you feel competitive with me. I want you to treat me as a real person," that he'd run from the house. I heard his voice angry from the bedroom after he had said a cursory goodnight to me. I heard him getting dressed and talking to Anna, "If she's standing out in the hall, I will beat the holy shit out of her."

I sat in the living room waiting, thinking I should leave by the side door and hide at the back of the house. Yet I wanted to go stand in the hall so as to dare him, to see if he would beat me, knowing from the time I had hit him that the one who strikes out feels guilt and remorse as well as relief, and in the end, the other one wins. I sat very still in the living room as he came out and loudly opened the front door. "I don't want to know about your feelings, you son-of-a-bitch," he yelled in at me as he left.

When he came back hours later, early into the morning, I took my calico cat in my arms and came out to sit across from him in the living room. Anna had knocked at my door and said he wanted to talk to me.

I told Marc that what I had wanted to say was, "I want you to love me." He replied that Anna had told him he might try being diplomatic with me, rather than passive or aggressive.

The next night we made an agreement about how we would talk to each other. Marc proposed a form full of blanks for use when either of us had something to say about what the other was doing wrong. I vowed I would never use the form. I would not appear dissatisfied, or chalk it up as the other guy's fault. As of yet, neither of us has used the procedure and Marc sometimes smiles at me.

Sometimes now, I imagine my father risen from the grave talking with Marc, taking a long walk with him, understanding him, patting him on the back and telling him he is a good man, that it will all work out. Marc should not let the world deal him blows. My father was less afraid of the world than Marc, but like Marc, he sought shelter in his home, his family. Like Marc, he was suspicious of me and some of my ways to power, and he always removed himself from what was clearly women's—from what transpired between my mother and me—as if he could not understand it.

At times, similarly, I see Marc disappearing into the hallway, not happy, I think, that Anna and I have words to mumble to each other alone. But I feel somehow this is fate. We cannot know one another's bonds. Yet we can allow those significant moments when those we love commune with those we do not understand, those whose existence we secretly wish to deny, for what it says about who we cannot be.

I will be a smaller child and a larger person than ever Marc was meant to know, and he will make a life with Anna while part of her heart reaches out toward me. He turns logs in the fire by poking at them with a stick. I, watching him, reach in with my bare hand, and grabbing a log by its non-burning end, slowly swivel it around. Marc is right, I do fight him. I am intent on showing him that I am, that I, too, have ingenuity, that I brave what he sometimes fears, what he may not even think to brave. I am sure I miss his courage, so intent am I on seeing my own. I miss his concessions to me, miss the importance of how he does care.

"Couldn't you get me a better father?" I asked Anna not long ago.

"I can teach him," she said. "But maybe it is wrong. Maybe I should accept what he cannot be."

We are each so large in the other's dreams, so important, so much more important than we are to ourselves.

"I love you, Anna. Perhaps I'll never love Marc."

"I don't like being a prize between you."

Anna and I fight more since Marc has come. One night last week, we argued and I drove off. When I returned to the house, I knocked at Anna's door. "What do you want?" she asked wearily as she opened it and followed me back to my room.

Inside, she stood near me. "I'm tired," she said. "You drain me. Won't you ever let me sleep?"

I felt scared and angry. I felt it was not right for me to want her. I picked up my wine glass from a table by my side and threw it across the room. Empty, it landed on the rug and did not break. I began hitting my leg with my fist. "Bad," I said of myself, "very bad."

"Stop it," Anna interrupted. Then she took me by the hand and led me to the bed and there she sat and held me as I sobbed.

"I don't want us to fight," I said to her. "I want to be littul, bery littul." Then I started making sucking noises with my mouth, took a piece of her nightgown between my lips and sucked at it until it was wet. "Tiny bebe, dat's me" and I cried again. I cried and cried until my crying became little laughs and Anna was laughing with me.

"Now go to sleep," she said finally. "Little babies need sleep," and I curled up on the bed then and she covered me, although I still had my clothes on.

The next morning, she told me that when she had gone back to her room that night, Marc was up. He said that he had been scared for me. Though months later, after he'd left, he told her he thought it had worked. When the two of them got close, I would have a fit and draw them apart. Then Anna would give in to me. That was how he lost her. It was all deliberate on my part, to get her to leave him, to send him away.

∞

For a while, Marc and I did get along. "I have problems with Anna," he said to me during that time, "but whatever happens, I want to be your friend." I did not respond except to say thank you, for fear that my saying I wanted the same would scare him. I so easily scared him.

One night, while the three of us sat watching television in the living room, I sat close to Marc and stroked his back. When I asked him to hold me, he did. The next day, he and I went for a walk. It was not as long as I would have liked and I sensed he wanted to come back to Anna. We did not talk "deep stuff" because I knew he would not want that. But we did go out together.

One evening, Anna stayed late at work and Marc and I were alone in the house. We made our separate dinners. Marc listened to records in the living room. I read books in my bedroom, and when I was done, brought a lamp out to him so he could see better while he was studying. Before he went to bed, I asked him into my room and told him about things that had happened to me in the day. He sat in the chair across from me rather stiffly, but he did lean forward and make an attempt to understand.

Another night when we had company, Marc got into an argument with the woman of the couple. Afterward, Anna was mad at him because on social occasions, he always fought stubbornly in an argument with someone. I felt I understood him since he was like me in arguing to assert himself. I went up to him and stroked his back and his neck. He said it felt good and calmed down. He acted like I was his friend.

A couple of months later, however, when I came back from spending a long weekend in California at a conference, the atmosphere had changed. Anna told me that she and Marc had fought over me while I was gone. Marc was sure I would never really leave.

I heard him the night I returned as I listened at their door. "She won't go," he said again and again. "I know she won't go."

"But I'm not her whole life, she has a job there."

"She'll turn it down."

"That's ridiculous."

"I'm not happy with you."

"I love you."

Earlier that day, I had gone into the kitchen and given Marc some special sponges he had asked for from California, and some wine and bread I had brought. Straight-faced at first, he finally smiled at me and said he was grateful. But soon, he announced he was going to bed. He walked determinedly out of the room. When he had left, Anna turned to me, "Don't try to reach out to him anymore. It hurts me to see you try so hard."

It was different from that time on, and I never accepted it. Marc spoke with small signs. When I came into a room, he stopped talking. He wanted dinner over fast so he and Anna could go into bed early. I would leave the door to my room open when I left the house; when I came back, I would always find it closed. He would enter and leave the house without saying hello or goodbye to me. When he went for a walk in the evening, he would take Anna's dog but not my puppy.

"You and Marc, you're alike," Anna said to me, "You don't feel that anyone cares that you're there."

"I can't stand her," Marc said to Anna of me. "She's absolutely controlling. Every move she makes is aimed at control."

"Is it Susan you can't stand, or is it that in yourself?"

"It's her. I told you. It's her."

Eventually I told Anna that I'd had desires to be sexual with Marc. She told me that she felt he loved me, even though he would never admit it. Once after Marc and I had fought and each apologized, he held me very tight. He always held me tight when he hugged me.

One night, he and Anna came back late from a party and Anna was very drunk. She had to lean on him to walk. I came out of my room and met them just inside the front door. I assumed Marc would undress Anna and help her to bed. Still, I had wanted to say goodnight to her. He nodded at me over her shoulder. "I'll tell you later," he said.

After he had put her to bed, he came out into the living room and sat with me. "I'm sorry," he began, "I know you wanted to talk to her."

"It can wait. I mostly wanted to say goodnight."

The two of us then talked about how we felt when Anna got drunk. "I get angry," I told him.

"At the party," he said, "she started drinking too much when they began talking about her mother. That was about three hours ago. She's been lost to us since then."

"You take care of her, you are good to her."

"I don't like to see her destroying herself."

"I can tell when I watch you and she decides to drink, I can tell you don't want to interfere."

"If I tell her no, she'll do it anyway," he said.

"You don't want her lost. You want to go to a party and be with her. Then drive home and talk about the evening. It must be hard on you."

"I know you're her friend. You wanted to see her."

That night after Marc had gone into bed, I bumped into a kitchen cabinet while I was making tea and dropped a large mug that was Anna's. It made a noise as it broke in pieces on the floor. Within moments, Marc came out. "I didn't do it on purpose," I told him, "it just dropped."

"Anna wants to see you. She wants to say goodnight. She's afraid you will be angry with her."

I went into the dark bedroom by myself then and leaned over the bed where Anna lay. She reached up her arms and pulled me to her. "Are you angry? Don't be angry with me," she said. "I'm bad, very bad."

"I was angry before, but Marc talked to me. I'm not mad anymore. You're not bad. Sometimes you get drunk because you don't want to face the things that disturb you."

She nodded and held me close, not wanting me to get up. I was worried that Marc would come in and see me in her arms and be hurt. After a while, he did come in and stood in the dark at the far end of the room: "I don't want to interrupt. I just wanted to know how long you'll be. So I'll know what to do."

"You're not interrupting, come be here with us," Anna said, still holding me.

He stood still in the doorway, unsure.

"Come," I looked toward him. "It's all right, it's not private."

He came then and lay down beside Anna on his side of the bed, looking over at her as she held me and talked as a little girl done wrong. He listened as I told her again and again that she was not bad, that there were more important things than her getting drunk. He listened as I joked with her and as she laughed.

"How are you feeling, honey?" she finally asked him, putting out an arm to touch his face.

"I'm okay. A little sad. I want Susan to be saying those things to me."

⌒⌒

Marc left four months after he moved in. I came home one night and found a bed and a chair missing from my room; they were his. Dishes and food from the night before lay out in the kitchen. The ashtrays in the living room were full, and usually he emptied them. Lights were on here and there, as if the house had been quickly abandoned. In Anna's bedroom, Marc's clothes were gone from the closet.

I was upset and I did not want to stay in the empty house. I drove off, leaving Anna a note, "Why didn't you warn me? Don't you care?"

When I returned, she was finally home. I walked into her bedroom and bent down to kiss her. Her lips did not move. "Are you angry with me?" I asked.

Anna sat up and looked at me blankly. "I want to be alone," she said. "I have feelings too, you know. Though probably you don't care. You overwhelm me with yours. You are so afraid, so very angry. You have lost your bed and your chair. I have lost my man."

Had she lost furniture, I might have been more understanding. Had she lost a child. But a man.

"Now get out," she said. "I want my privacy. Can't you leave me alone? I am asking you—let me have my tragedy."

I stood there not moving, shaken. "I didn't mean—"

"I don't care what you meant. I didn't know he was going to leave tonight. I didn't know what he had taken. I came home from work early and he was pulling out in a truck. I hate you. Can you hear that? Leave me alone. I'll talk to you in a week."

I left her room, slamming the door behind me. Then I drove off in my car for the second time that night. The next morning when I came into the kitchen, Anna was already up, and I was unsure of how to behave with her. I put on the pot for coffee and stepped wide of her. There were long silences between our words. When she left the house, I wished her a good day.

Later, she called me from work to say she was okay, to ask how I was, to ask about earrings she wanted to get as presents for friends, to tell me she had gone to two stores and become confused. I told her I would help her, that it was hailing out at the house, we were having a storm like I had never seen.

That evening when I met Anna in town, I told her I was sorry for my behavior the night before, and I cried as I said it. When we came back to the house that night, the rooms were strange in their darkness, for had Marc been there, lights would have been on. The floors in the living room and kitchen were clean and they had been dirty before I left. "Marc has left you a present," I said to Anna, motioning to them.

We sat in the living room eating a dinner I felt Anna did not want to eat, as if, why bother, since Marc was gone. Soon she became tearful. "My old man," she said, "he moves out and he comes back to clean my floors."

I wished then that I had cleaned them, that I had not told her it was his work, and we talked of other things. When I kissed her goodnight, she kissed me back.

The next day Anna spent with Marc. They went to a party and then to his new house. The morning after that, when I woke, Anna told me of it and of how Marc had blamed his moving out on me. He had been telling her for weeks that I was forcing him out, I controlled her life, took over the house. When her son came to visit her next month, I would push him out too. I would not let her date. No man would come near her because of how I would act. And she, he said, she would respond as she always had, by taking care of me.

Anna did take care of me, I knew, though perhaps not in the way Marc thought. She and I now began to live alone in the house again, though differently than we had before. All that had happened was there with us. We talked in the mornings and late at night, each day a little more easily. Yet it would be a while before I would see Anna without hearing the words of the others—Marc and Anna's brother and people she met at parties, who said, because they had spoken with Marc, "How hard it must be to live with a third person." How hard, especially, because that person is the kind she is.

After Marc left, Anna became more afraid. "I don't know if I can make it without him," she said.

I looked at her with eyes that did not know what to make of what I saw. I did not know how hard the time between us would become, how very tired she would soon be, how necessary it would be to start over, as if the split, when Marc left, was with me, not him.

After Marc moved out, I cleaned the refrigerator. It reminded me of an earlier time when I had cleaned it soon after I had moved in. Though then I did not know that the orange juice I was throwing out had been there since he had left the spring before, or that was Anna's recollection. Now I knew that the four dried-out hot dogs I disposed of were from a package that had made him sick two weeks back; the onions were ones he had chopped a month ago; the stale turkey and fermented dressing remnants of the last dinner we had cooked for three.

Marc is gone now, but his mail still comes to the mailbox sometimes and I pick it up and don't know what to do with it. I want to give it back, tell people at the post office not to send it anymore. But I bring it home and leave it on the counter in the kitchen for Anna, who still sees him. I look for his car all the time. It doesn't matter if the roads I travel are nowhere near where he might be. I imagine him still in the house sometimes. Yet I don't tell Anna because she has told me that she wants her own grief. She does not like me taking it away.

I did not want Marc living here and I didn't want him to go. I never believed he would leave before I would. Late the night he moved out, before I went to sleep, after Anna and I had been at odds, I came out to the living room and looked at the basket of peanuts he had left on top of the television and took them quickly and put them in the cupboard in the kitchen. I did not want Anna to see them in the morning and be sad.

IV: IF WE WERE FREE

I came home early in the evening in a borrowed truck with two chairs Anna had bought the day before. She came out of the house to help me unload them. I got up inside the truck bed and handed the chairs down to her one at a time, first the bentwood rocker, then the basket chair. We brought them into the living room and placed them near the fireplace, below pictures on the far wall. They sat there and glowed, almost like two people, especially the rocker with its blonde wood.

"I was afraid of bringing them back," I had told Anna when I first arrived. "I feared you would not like them, that I would be like a messenger with bad news."

She shook her head, as if unsure of where such an idea might have come from. "They're perfect. They're just what I wanted," she said.

"And your medicine, I brought that too."

"You are good to me." She stepped close to where I stood beside the truck. "You look happy," she said, in a way that surprised me, parting the neck of my shirt. "You've a little sunburn, I see."

Soon Anna went to plant the flowers we had also bought the day before. They had sat in the garage and were beginning to wilt. While she was out in the garden, Marc called and I went to fetch her. When she came in, she made a date with him for dinner for an hour later, for first she wanted to finish planting the flowers. I went out and knelt to help her, to dig little holes she might fill with seedlings. The air was clear and becoming cool. A huge moon stood in the blue-gray sky, and beyond it were the mountains and high silver clouds.

"It feels good to be out and planting now," I said.

"Yes, it does."

We were happy together.

When we finished the planting, Marc came. I had not expected him to appear at the house. I had not seen him since he moved out. I had thought Anna would drive down to the restaurant to meet him. Yet suddenly he stood there in the doorway to the kitchen. I was making toast and I did not want to leave the room. I heard Anna say hello to him and ask about his trip. They dealt with each other cautiously. There was no hug. They stood in the doorway talking. I moved to the stove to fetch a pot I wanted to wash to use for cooking my dinner, so I would have something to do without leaving the room. I wanted Marc to deal with me and, at the same time, I was very scared. I had almost stopped breathing when he walked in. I had looked at his head and it seemed very big. He had not said hello to me, so finally I turned from the sink and said it to him.

He looked up surprised. "Hello," he said, as if I could not matter less. Then he went to the bedroom to look for a painting he had forgotten to take. Anna showed him her new chairs. Before she left, she came to me in the kitchen and kissed me. "Thank you," she said. "I love you."

As she walked out with Marc, I wished her a good time. Later, I made my dinner, spoke on the phone with friends, and finally went to bed. Yet I lay wide awake thinking. I did not expect Anna back before I slept. I imagined she would go to Marc's apartment after dinner and stay with him late. Thus when car lights pulled into the drive, they surprised me. I heard Anna open the front door, heard her talking to the dogs, her voice calm and friendly. I heard the water running in the kitchen sink and the pot begin to boil for tea. I wanted to come out right away to see her but stopped myself. She might need to be alone after leaving Marc. I did not want to see the wistful expression on her face that would speak of her feelings for him, to feel her home but in another world. I wanted her to knock on my door and come in and find me.

Finally, I got out of bed, wrapped a blanket around myself, and walked out into the hall. I met Anna in the doorway to the kitchen. She seemed glad to see me. "I thought you were asleep," she said.

"I was trying, but I'm wide awake."

"Come in and talk to me on my bed," she gestured with her mug. "I'm making tea."

I walked back into my room to change my blanket for a nightgown and sat for a while on my bed, listening to her noises, wanting not to come out before she had gone to the toilet and undressed. I went into my bathroom, combed my hair, and looked at my face in the mirror, waiting. Then Anna was at my door in her nightgown. "Are you coming?" she asked.

I followed her out, across the hall, and into her room. On her bed, I sat beside her. She seemed happy and I felt glad. For I had not expected her invitation, or that she would come to see if I was ready.

"Did you have a good time?" I asked.

"I had a very good time. I have a good time with Marc now that we see each other this way."

She described the restaurant in which they had eaten: the food, how some of it was Jewish food, with that kind of fish in white sauce.

"Herring?"

"Yes."

Then she told me she thought she would spend the night after next with Marc. She would not come home.

"Does that mean you're becoming sexually involved with him?" I asked.

"Yes, it does." She looked at me, waiting.

I was suddenly afraid and began to cry. "When you become sexually involved with someone, with a man, with Marc, I think I'll always feel, 'why couldn't it be me?'"

"Wouldn't it be worse if it were a woman?"

I thought a moment. "Yes."

"It won't be a woman."

"To comfort myself, I think of what it would be like between you and me, even if that would never happen, that it would be different." My voice started to break.

Then the dogs, who had been lying at the foot of Anna's bed— my puppy and Anna's larger, silvery gray dog—suddenly went to the window, growling. I wished not to hear, not to notice the interruption. Anna sat up very straight, alert, turning to the window.

"It sounds like horses," I said.

"I'm afraid," she looked at me, then out the window once more. "The dogs don't usually act like this."

There were sounds again and I thought it was a man running. Then definitely, I heard a horse. I imagined a rider going back and forth by the house, a crazy man. Next the noise sounded out front, by the kitchen. The man was circling the house.

Anna got out of bed. "I'm afraid," she said again, and we walked together down the hall toward the kitchen.

"If we see him, I'll call the neighbors for help," I offered.

I checked the front door, found it locked, then walked into the living room and turned the key in the door there. Anna looked out the kitchen window. "It's the baby," she said quietly after a moment, "from next door, and the mother. They must have gotten out."

I dialed the neighbors with the number already in my hand, told them their horses were out, the mother and the filly. They said they would be right over. They did not want them to run away. I came out into the living room, looked past Anna's shoulder through the window and saw the two horses there in the dark: the baby coming close on the cement patio just outside the glass door, the mother near, munching on weeds. Then a third head—the male horse, too, was out.

"They're all out," I said to Anna. "They'll come get them. They thanked me for calling."

She motioned me back to the bedroom to get a robe in case the neighbors knocked on the door. "I don't want to be in here," she said, meaning the bedroom, where the light was on. "They might see us sitting here talking."

I followed her back out to the hall. "We can sit in the dark in the living room," I said.

"Come," she led me to a corner of the kitchen. "Let's sit here."

We sat down on the floor in the corner on a little rug where we used to sit at night in the winter when the house was too cold, near the one heater that blew very hot. We sat in the dark, I beside Anna at an angle to her so I could see her face. She held her mug of tea and reached for an ashtray and her cigarettes. My puppy jumped up suddenly and knocked over her ashtray. She got up to take a towel and wipe the floor. When she sat again, I was nervous, waiting. The light from the front hallway illuminated her face. Her eyes glowed intensely. I expected she would want to talk about the horses and of our fears. But instead she sought to continue our earlier conversation.

"If we were free," I began, fighting my tears, "it might be very tender, special. I want to know if you feel that way too."

"Yes," she said after a pause, looking off into space, thinking, taking a puff on her cigarette, but I did not believe her.

"I don't want to be the manipulative child," I said. "I can take care of myself, no matter what you do. But I get afraid that your body will draw you away. If you become sexually involved with Marc, with anyone, that will be the most compelling thing in your life."

She looked to her side and up toward the window, where a breeze was coming in. "It was that way with you." She paused, began again.

"I still think of you in the day. When I'm at work on those long days. I don't call you. I don't call anyone. But I think of you a lot."

"Back then, when you first had those feelings for me," I said, "I felt affirmed, like a whole person, your equal. It was a way for me to be close with you and not be in the role of a child. I felt like a full human being, a real woman."

She looked toward the window again, then turned to me. "I betrayed you then, with what I did."

"You didn't. I didn't feel it as betrayal."

"I did. I betrayed you."

"I get afraid now that because you won't be sexual with me, you'll turn me into a child every time we get close."

"I don't always turn you into a child. These past two weeks, you've been a woman for me often."

Then I told her of my more basic fear. "I feel I hate Marc, but I know it's not him. It's me. I'm afraid now to be alone at night. I think it's the loss of a dream, or of a sense of security I had in the thought that every night, you'd come home to me. No matter what else you would do, you'd come home."

"I do come home."

"But the ritual, the reliability. You've been here every night since I moved in, except for Thanksgiving when you went to see Marc."

When I next looked over at Anna, she was again looking past me, her eyes filling with tears.

"What are you feeling?" I asked.

"What you say about my not coming home, that's how I've felt about Marc being gone."

"What else?"

"Despair. I felt sad when you told me about your pain, but I didn't feel like crying until I thought of the betrayal. I betrayed you when I became sexual with you. Our agreement was for you to be like a child to me. I was to give you a different kind of experience. Then I acted like all the others. I betrayed you then."

"You didn't betray me. I never wanted our relationship to be defined strictly as mother-child."

"I know."

"Maybe you betrayed something within yourself."

Yet I knew that Anna always wanted that simpler relationship, in which sex was not acted upon, or not felt. She would refer to it time and again in moments of regret, of apology, of feeling that all else between us that was not mother-child or distant friend was wrong. And always this hurt me and seemed untrue. It was not how we were.

"Maybe someday," I said to her, "Maybe a few years from now, I'll know the value of what you are telling me and be thankful." I looked at her face, seeking to reassure her, to find there what was right. I wanted to believe that all our struggles, all my difficulty in accepting the lines she had to draw, would in the end be worth the effort. I wanted to let her teach me, to let her lead. For I would have led, even that night, with a kiss, a gentle hand that might have ended with us, for moments, in an uneasy passion.

"What else do you feel?" I asked.

"I feel exhausted."

I thought a moment. "Will you hold me now, as a child?"

"I don't want to treat you as a child tonight," she said. "You have been a woman in how you've spoken with me. I want to respond to the woman."

I feared then for the child, for that part of myself that needed comfort, safety. I saw myself rising and going off to bed, heard our separate doors shut.

"No. Respond to the child," I said. "I was good. I was a woman, and the reward for me is to be at last held as a child."

"I can't do that," she looked at me sadly, very tired. "You sat and talked with me tonight, you didn't throw things or break things like you used to. You gave me space, you told me of your feelings, but you didn't demand that I change. You said you could take care of yourself."

She stood up then and reached a hand down to me. I took it and rose at her side. She put her mug and ashtray on the counter behind her and we embraced. I felt her body close against mine, her head at my cheek. "You're right," I said, "I'm a woman tonight." For it was being held that I'd wanted, woman or child did not matter. I felt, in her arms, the comfort I had sought with my questions and words. The shut doors disappeared.

"I should have asked you to hold me sooner," I said as I drew back from her and she looked into my eyes, her own frank and open, fully there. Her eyes scared me. She was looking at me as a woman. I felt the strength, the depth of the commitment, her feeling for me.

And then it was I who pulled away as we turned to walk down the hall to our bedrooms. I lapsed into child talk, speaking to myself in a way that is quick and makes words small.

"Not child tonight," Anna said.

"Yes child. When I'm happy, I am child."

I did not know then to say, or even think, that I might be feeling like a child because I was afraid, afraid of that moment when our eyes had met and I had felt, in Anna's gaze, the reward for being a woman, the acknowledging of a fullness in me I had not felt was my own, that I feared would not last.

Anna went to the bathroom, then came into my bedroom to say goodnight. She reached out her hand toward me. "You and I are finding new ways of being," she said, and her gaze was steady, searching. I wanted not to meet it, not to scare her away. I looked quickly at her, then down.

After she left my room, I walked out into the kitchen and looked at the clock; it was two. Anna and I had not stayed up that late for a very long time. I came back into my room and lay down, but I could not sleep. I took up a pen and paper and started to write—a long note that would allow me to cry, to continue a conversation I never wanted stopped: "Anna, I'm afraid you'll push me too fast before I'm ready. Anna . . ."

Much later, I walked out to the kitchen and put a briefer note on the chopping block where Anna would see it in the morning. The sky was beginning to get light. The sun was coming up. Anna had always told me I should see the sunrise over the distant mountains. I had seen it one morning when I lay in bed with her. She woke me and I had buried my head. "Not again," I said, "unless it's before I go to sleep."

I stood in the kitchen now, tired yet alert, poured myself a glass of wine, and waited a few minutes for the sun. It was not ready. I took the glass and the wine bottle and walked back to my room, stumbling. I wondered if women did this, drank themselves to sleep. I turned out the lights and lay in bed, waiting for the wine to take effect. From my bedroom window, I could see the sky beginning to turn pink. I thought I should go out and check again for the sun, to see it finally rise over the mountains, and then I began to cry. I sobbed. I heard my puppy rustling in his bed outside my bedroom door. I thought that he had heard me, and I wished that Anna had, though the walls between us were thick.

I sobbed with anger. I fought with my father, I beat at him with my fists, cursed my mother for holding onto an ideal vision of him after he died. I cursed her for being so beautiful, so enticing to me. I cried loudly until I slept.

In the morning when I woke, my head was thick with a hangover, my eyes swollen, my body shaking, and I still cried. Hours passed before my head became bearable and my body, while no longer shaking, began to get unstuck. I went into the kitchen. Anna had gone but had left me a note: "I want the woman to grow, and I will protect and hold the child. I love you."

I drank coffee. When I left the house, I put on dark glasses, for the sun outside was too bright. I felt like maybe it was a new day. Yet I was no longer feeling the comfort of being a woman that I had felt the night before. I was simply no longer feeling.

Standing outside the house, I looked over my shoulder and saw the horses now safely in their pens. I was very tired and climbed into the borrowed truck to take it back and marveled that it moved.

Twice, I nearly ran it off the road. I so wanted it to be a new day, a day of excitement, of my being, at last, what I wished. Yet somewhere I knew I was not ready. It would be a while before I would meet Anna's eyes with the assurance I needed.

∽

Anna was about to go out with Marc again. She came in to say good-night to me before she left. "I'm angry," I said to her as we sat on my bed. "You're fooling yourself."

"I want you to love me. I may foul up my life. But I want you to love me anyway." She looked at me with tears in her eyes.

A few nights later, Anna and I were watching television, a program in which the lead man had a cleft in his chin, as have all the men in Anna's life—her father, her husband, the men she has dated, Marc, her sons. "If you weren't a woman, you'd still have a problem with me," she said, "because you don't have a cleft in your chin."

"I'm trying," I told her, putting my finger to my chin, pushing hard.

"I don't know if I'll ever be as happy as I've been with you," she added as I turned to go out to the kitchen.

"It hasn't all been happiness. You've had a lot of trouble with me."

"I've been happy often."

The following evening, she came home with a bagful of groceries in her arms, determined to go on a diet. She was going to exercise. She wanted to give up drinking and smoking, to change her life style.

We sat on the couch in the living room, and she spoke of the new life she planned: "I want to eat only healthy foods. You know the feeling, that nothing you put into your body is bad. In a few months, you won't recognize me. I'll be thin, like I used to be. Maybe I won't drink for four or five months. I'll have to find something else to do. When I come home, I can't watch TV and sit talking, or I'll want a drink. Maybe I should take a bath."

"Then get into bed?" I asked her.

"Yes, I'd like that."

"You look sad," she said to me after a while, noticing my eyes.

"I am. I cry a lot in the days. It's not anything you've done. It's what's going on inside of me. I'm determined to be good, not to hold onto you, or anyone, out of fear that they'll abandon me. It's moving to me, how I try, that I might do it. So I cry."

When I went into Anna's room later to say goodnight, the pills I had taken for my headache affected me and I was slow, as in a dream. It was easier to say goodnight with the pills. I put my head to her breast and she kissed me and there was no talk of my being a child.

The next evening, Anna came home earlier than I had expected. I was in her bathroom running a bath for her, about to measure some oil to pour in. I had lit two candles and they were sitting by the sink, with the ceiling light still on. In her bedroom, I had drawn down the covers, turned on the lamp beside the bed, and opened the windows. I wanted her to come home and be cared for, feel special. In the midst of my drawing the bath, the front door opened. I turned around and she was suddenly behind me.

"A bath?"

"Your bath. You weren't supposed to be home yet."

We had dinner that night on Anna's bed and spoke of the day. I told her I was planning to tune my car. Before he left, Marc had advised me that I should know how to do it since I wanted to buy a VW van and they threw rods all the time. I had bought the parts. It would be the first time I had tuned a car and if it worked, I would be proud.

Anna told me of the place where she had gone to exercise earlier that day. She had pulled on machines, though the meter never registered her strength. She had met some men: "That's where they are. I went in and they flocked around me right away."

"I was afraid of that," I said. "One night you won't come home. But it's good. I'm glad for you."

Of the men she had met, "One of them was Marc's age," she said. And from this I was to gather what she meant: that Marc's age, seven years younger than hers, was intriguing—young enough to be imaginable as her child. For the orphans, always the orphans, spoke to her, those whose mothers had died, who had left them too young. Yet she wanted, I knew, an older man who would take her in, who would hold her in his heart and not only in bed. I wanted to be that man. I wanted it very much.

"Anna, I want to be larger than your life."

"You already are."

"But I mean in a different way."

"You are."

"Anna, do you think I am a woman?" I asked her later that night, when I came in to say goodnight and give her a last kiss.

"Yes, I think you are a woman, a golden one."

I looked into her eyes.

"I heard two songs on the radio today," she said. "They were sad songs, sung by one woman to another, songs of loss, that the one had lost a woman she loved."

I shook my head, disbelieving. The station was not one to play such songs.

"You know how to please me," she said.

"You are not hard to please."

"You don't think so. Other people do."

"You are easy to please."

She shook her head, and her gaze was remote, fastening on some other pleasure, I thought, some missed dream, Marc. But for the moment, because she was with me, and because we were here, safe on her bed, I was happy. I did not tell this to Anna, however, fearing my happiness would break, fearing the time between us, so fine when removed and in its own little world, would be short-lived.

When I went back into my room that night, I was less fearful than in a long time. Anna would seek new men and I would be the one who stayed home, who was home more than Anna or I even knew. The house was hers, but I stayed there days. I worked there, I wrote, I did shopping, I cooked. I saw to it that garbage did not accumulate. I fed the dogs and took care of my cat. Somewhere in me was this basic desire to be wife, and in Anna, the desire to be given rest, to come home from a day and find me there, as if I had never left.

When finally I would leave, she would miss me, I thought. She would miss me as ground from beneath her feet, although she had said I was "fire," not "ground." Marc was ground. I was, I knew, both. If I could make a home, if I could be home to her, I could be this for myself, I thought. I would not wander lost as I had been.

For when I first met Anna, I was quite lost, between jobs, between homes. When I moved into her house, Marc had not been there, although he had been in her life. At first, I had asked Anna's permission each time I used the washing machine. I did not know how to take care of a dog, or how to leave Anna's bed after I said goodnight. Back then, I was careful of Anna because of what I did not know about her.

Now we knew each other better. Anna knew what would speak to my fears. The next morning when she left the house, she left me a note: "I love you. Take care of yourself, and I'll be back."

It was the last phrase that spoke to me most especially. For it used to be that when she went out or I left, Anna would say to me, "Have fun. Have a good time." I would tell her I'd see her later. After a while, she came to know that what I wanted to hear was that she would return, or that she would be there when I came home. She, on the other hand, wished to be told to have fun, for this was what her mother had not done. Her mother had sat up at night crying, waiting for her to come home.

I was out in the garage late the next morning working on my car. I had just removed a part and I was worried that I had not replaced it properly. "Anna," I came out to find her reading at the kitchen counter, still in her nightgown. "I'm scared," I said as I sank to the floor at her feet, sitting where we had huddled that night the horses got out. "I'm afraid the car won't work. I wish the old part was still there. Can you come step on the gas for me?"

She looked down at me smiling. "We are each so afraid," she said. "You're afraid of your car. I'm afraid of my life."

I stood up and she hugged me. Then she picked up her mug of tea, followed me out to the garage, and there, as if enacting some ancient drama, we made sure the car, lurching slightly, could at least function enough to get me to a gas station.

That night, Anna read her book in the living room and I sat near her and wrote. Soon she went into bed and I went to lie with her.

"I'm thinking of getting a dog," she said, "a big one who will bark and scare people. For after you leave. A female."

I was shocked. Could I be so easily replaced? "I love you very much," I said.

"I love you too."

Part Two

Feeling Illicit

V: FAMILY VISITS

The latch on the front gate clicked. Anna's son Timothy had arrived. Anna stood from where we were sitting in the living room and went to the door to greet him, giving him a long hug. I stayed behind, shuffling magazines, then went out also and gave him a hug, but shorter. That evening, after Anna and Tim had spent time talking, we moved a bed from the garage into the other half of Anna's large bedroom, and Timothy went in to lie down and read.

Anna stood with me in the kitchen. "You're in shock," she said, and I shook my head, wanting to think differently. "He has finally come. Things will change for you again."

Yet I did not really feel they had changed until I went to bed myself and could no longer go into Anna's room and give her one last kiss. I put the dogs out in the hall and closed my bedroom door. I would weather this one, I thought. I liked Tim.

He had come from California in his truck with a trailer he had made chained to it, a small wooden houselike structure with a shingled roof which he said caught attention as he drove. In it he carried his motorcycle, his bike, two large crates of tools, a stereo, beer, and a very scared cat who followed him into the house and hid in corners. Tim, twenty-one, was Anna's youngest and quite handsome, his face, his gentleness, reminiscent of hers. He was the one she felt she had left too soon when she moved here from California after her own mother died three years ago. He would stay for two months and Anna had a list of work for him to do: repairing windows, refinishing furniture, pulling weeds, planting in the garden. As she went through all she'd planned for him, he smiled over at me. His mom, we both somehow understood, was, at times, impossible; she wanted to do too much. Yet this sharing, his smile, was so different from what I had felt with Marc that I was reassured.

I offered Tim some dinner that I was making; Anna did too. But he declined. He wanted to take care of himself, he said.

Tim had not known that Marc had gone. Anna told him minutes after he arrived. "So it's just the two of you and me," he said.

"And two cats and two dogs," I added.

The next day, about midmorning, Marc called and I answered. Anna was out, so he asked to talk with Timothy. Tim took the phone in my room, sat on the floor in front of me, and I listened. Marc was asking him about going camping, going to the races, spending time. When Tim hung up, he turned to me. "Marc's a neat guy," he said.

I looked at him, for I had been waiting. "Marc blames his moving out on me," I said. "He may say bad things about me. I don't want you to hate me because of what he says."

Timothy lay back on the floor, took one of my puppy's toys, and started teasing him with it. This was his answer as I sat there lost in the weight of my words, my seriousness.

"I listen to everyone and take a little bit of what each one says," he finally replied, looking up at me thoughtfully.

That evening while Anna and I were preparing dinner, she made a remark, in Timothy's hearing, about my being controlling, that Marc had felt it, that it was true. I became angry and did not want to look at her. I sat at the table with Anna and Timothy and I was very quiet. After dinner, when Tim had gone to bed, Anna and I argued in the kitchen, things long simmering between us coming to the surface. I told her I did not like being called controlling. She called me a "manipulative, demanding child." I told her she was a queen, lording it over everyone. She said what was wrong was all my fault. I said with two people, it had to be half and half.

As we walked down the hallway toward our bedrooms, our words were still angry and we whispered them so Timothy would not hear. Yet somehow, in those moments of arguing, things seemed to get better. I kissed Anna and said that I loved her. She said she loved me too.

The next morning before Anna left for work, she sat on the floor in the corner of the kitchen, nervous, beginning to cry. "I'm not happy," she said. "I don't think I'll ever be happy."

I bent down to speak to her, to reassure her, aware of Tim standing by, that he would overhear, wondering how often he had seen his mother like this, worried for what he would think of my words: "It's a hard time for you. It won't always be this way. Next year at this time, you'll be happier."

She got up soon, gathering her things from the counter, preparing to leave. As she and Tim stood by the front door, I smiled at her, and over her shoulder at Tim. "Timothy will make you happy."

"We'll get some things done, some things finished," he turned to her, nodding, looking down from his height. "I'll do the yard, plant grass. You'll feel better then."

That day, Tim began working in the yard, digging a trench, bringing railroad ties to build a wall that would separate the yard from the surrounding desert landscape. I stayed in my room and typed.

In the evening, Anna came home early. We all had dinner and Tim and I joked. Two children, I thought. We will fill her life with children. I felt at one with Tim, yet wanted not to, not to be so simply or clearly Anna's child.

I heard Timothy and Anna in their bedroom later that night, talking and laughing behind the closed door, as I used to do with

Anna before sleep. I wanted to be the one who was there. But I did not feel as badly as I had when Marc was here.

After they were asleep, I went into the kitchen and made a salad for Anna to take to work the next day. I put it, with two apples, a fork, and a napkin, in a bag in the refrigerator, then left her a note saying it was there.

In the morning when I woke, she had already gone and left me a note in reply. "You are very good to me," it said.

During Tim's second week, he came down with a fever. I found him a doctor, gave him directions on how to bring down the fever, took his temperature, went out to the store to buy orange juice and magazines. He was sick all day. I stayed around working, feeling good—strong and sane somehow.

When Anna came home that evening, she came into my room to thank me. "You are truly my friend," she said. "You are a gift." I felt warmed, appreciated.

Another evening, after Tim had gone to bed early, his body sore and tired from the work he had done outside, Anna and I sat up together talking in the living room like we used to. On those nights when she and I talked and had a good time together, I did not stay up late or leave her notes for the morning. Yet the other nights when we were apart were in my mind still and I asked her about them a few days later, those nights when I kept waiting. "It starts before dinner," I told her, "especially when I'm alone. I get very sad. I want to lie down and not do anything."

"What do you think you are waiting for?" she asked.

"My mother. For my mother to come and take care of me."

For several nights after, I said to myself, "Stop waiting, stop waiting for mother," and it seemed to help.

Yet I waited nonetheless, for Anna, all too aware of how her presence seemed to center my life. I felt steady and not sad when I took care of her, or Tim. I had a purpose. There were rewards. And the more Anna was gone, as she was in those weeks after Timothy came—to classes early in the morning, staying late at work—the more I filled the spaces she left with small ways of taking care. I ignored her hesitations: "I don't want you to do things for me and then later be mad." Instead I responded to the asking I saw in her face, the relief when something she had not had time to do was done.

I cleaned the fireplace in the living room, and painted it white, washed and waxed the red tile floors, did laundry, made sure the counters in the kitchen were clear, took the spread from Anna's bed and had it cleaned, ran errands, cooked. I did my own work of typing and writing, but I also watched and waited. I waited for something new to begin, something old to be over.

One weekend as Anna and I sat talking at the dining table, she reached across and took my hand. "There's no one who understands me as you do," she said, looking at me with moist eyes. Then suddenly, the phone rang, interrupting us. It was her brother's wife. I heard her making plans to spend an evening at her brother's with Timothy and with her daughter, who would soon arrive, and with Marc; then an evening, a dinner, at our house, which Anna later told me I could not attend. For her brother had said he would not come if I was there. In his eyes, I was too important, too controlling in her life, and, in addition, we disagreed about politics.

I had wanted to be part of Anna's family. Yet I was some sort of bastard daughter, an illicit friend.

Anna had tried to tell me one evening that there were things I did not understand. I was a homosexual and I did not expect to pay for it. I expected that because the people who knew me loved me, all others would. I was not prepared when this worked against me.

"I know. I am not naive," I said.

But repeatedly she shook her head.

"It's not the people who don't know me I fear," I told her, "but the ones who seem to be close." I was thinking of Marc, fighting some private war with him still. "There are people who know me in personal ways, who feel I am a manipulator. In the back of their minds, there's a stereotype and it's going all the time. They don't see me. They think that I want to go to bed with their wife, that I'll steal their women friends. They see me as controlling you. These are the people that hurt me."

"No, you're not thinking," Anna was now sitting erect on the couch. "Listen, you're not hearing what I'm telling you."

Some nights later, I was reading in my room when car lights shone brightly in the driveway. I heard a knock on the front door. Anna was back; she was coming home after having had dinner at her brother's with Marc and Tim. She had forgotten her keys. I opened the door and Marc came into the house behind her. When I saw him, I stepped back and retreated toward my room. In the hallway outside my bedroom door, I heard Anna telling Timothy in the kitchen that she would be going back to Marc's apartment to spend the night.

"I thought you guys had split up," Tim said.

"We live in different houses," she answered him, laughing, and Marc joined her. "But we don't really know what's going on."

She laughed again and I knew she was quite drunk. When I had first come out to open the door for her, she had immediately put her arms around me and kissed me in that free way that said that drink had gone to her head. Seeing Marc behind her, I had somehow known before it was said. This would be Anna's first night staying over with Marc since he had moved out.

Anna came into my room to say goodbye to me. I was sitting on the end of my bed, silent. She sat down next to me and put her arms around me. "Tell me you'll still love me," she said.

"I'll still love you."

Then she went back out to join Marc. I heard her laughter as she closed the front door, as if this were the eve of some illicit celebration. She and Marc called in goodnights to Tim and he wished them a good time.

After they were gone, I went into Tim's bedroom and asked him if he would talk to me. I sat down on his bed across from him. "I get upset," I told him, "when she does this. I don't like it when she's drunk, that she has to get so drunk to go."

He paused for a moment before he answered: "The way I look at it is it's their business. I don't interfere. Marc's a great guy. He was happy tonight, and Mom was happy. You shouldn't let it get to you.

"Marc may be a great guy. But I don't think he's good for your mother. He moved out for a reason. He doesn't meet her needs, she's told me."

"All the men she's been with. She's always fought with them. She's always wanted to change them. She fought with my dad. I didn't like it. I don't get involved anymore. My dad couldn't accept when my sister got married. He wouldn't talk to her for months, but then he came around."

"Are you saying that Marc will come around to me?"

"Yeah."

"But this is different—"

Suddenly Anna was back, at the front door, upset. She'd had a fight with Marc, she said. "I told him to take me home if he was going to fight with me."

She walked hurriedly into the kitchen. "I'm going to make tea. Do you want some?" she called out to Tim. "Do you want crackers?"

"Was the fight about me?" I asked her, following her into the kitchen.

"It always is."

"Do you think I'm the reason he left?" I asked her then, wanting Tim to hear, to hear it from her.

"I don't. But Marc does. He is totally irrational when it comes to you. He hates you and there's nothing you can do about it."

She drank her tea, then called Marc and asked him to pick her up, making him swear not to fight with her again and to get her back first thing in the morning. Marc arrived and she left again.

Tim and I continued our talk.

"I don't trust your mom when she's drunk," I told him. "I don't trust she's rational."

"I do," he said. "Mom has always gotten drunk. I don't like it that she drinks. Just like I don't like it that she smokes. But I don't think she's irrational. When she drinks, she doesn't have the control over her emotions she usually has. Her emotions come out more. But she knows what she's doing. Mom always knows what she's doing. I trust her. She's always been there for me. My mom has been very good to me. She's always helped me, over all the years." He lay back in his bed. "I owe her a lot. She's always been very good to me. Even when I've done things she doesn't like."

After we finished talking, I went back into my room and lay awake for hours, angry, crying, afraid, wishing to break things, to storm about in rage, to pick up the phone and dial Marc's number, let it ring and then suddenly hang up. I lay in bed shaking, my hands at my sides, wishing I could be like Tim, seeing the room spin 'round and 'round, wanting to run, to escape, holding my chest tight, fighting it, feeling I had on a straightjacket which was binding my arms. The wine I tried to drink tasted bad. The scene was silly, I thought. Tim was right, I should not let it upset me. This was Anna's first night away; there would be others, and she would be back. Yet I was not Tim and I shook and cried and waited and no mother came to take care of my child. Though at last, near sunrise, I fell asleep.

I visited more with friends during those weeks, watched television more when I was alone, and waited.

VI: NO MODEL FOR OUR KIND

The day before Anna's daughter came to visit, I returned to the house and found Marc sitting in the living room, helping Anna with her statistics. I took a glass of wine and sat on the couch across from them, mostly silent. Finally, I said some words to Anna, whereupon Marc stood quickly, gave her a kiss and left.

"I wanted to look at him," I told her later. But she did not seem to want an explanation.

"You turn them away," she said to me, referring to Marc and her brother.

"I do not. It's your relationship with me they can't stand."

"It's a sick relationship."

"It's not."

"Yes it is."

"I don't control you."

"You do."

We drove off from the house then, each in our separate cars. When we came back, nothing was settled. We were still arguing, standing in the kitchen. At one point, Anna came toward me with a plastic milk carton raised over her head, as if to hit me with it. "I want to kill you," she whispered, so Timothy would not hear. "I will not have my son exposed to this."

"He's a grown man. He can take care of himself."

"You're lucky he doesn't turn away from you too."

"He and I have a relationship."

"I don't trust you in the house with him. There's no telling what you'll do."

Anna's daughter Janice came the next day. She asked that her mother not work the week of her visit, knowing Anna's way of easily feeling pulled in too many directions.

I heard Anna on the phone that afternoon telling a friend that her daughter had come, and that she and Marc were getting along beautifully, they only lived in different houses. I heard her making plans for spending time with Marc and her children during Janice's visit. Quietly I sat by myself in my room and drank wine and wanted to leave for California sooner than I had planned. It all made sense, I felt. Anna was with me one minute. "You are so important to me," she would say. "You understand me better than anyone else in the world. You are a gift." And then she was gone—to spend the night with Marc, or with her family. She was with me and then she would be gone.

That evening, I asked her into my room and told her I wanted to leave for California a month early, that I was having too much pain.

"I'm angry with you," she responded. "You'll be running away. It's always your pain. Don't you think about me? How do you think I'll feel if you go?"

We stood physically apart, a long silence between us. Then she came close and put her arms around me, where I stood rigid with my intention to leave.

In the next few days, I changed my mind and decided to stay until the end of the summer. I did not pick up the packing boxes I had ordered at the liquor store. I had needed to be asked, to be told I was wanted.

We managed through Anna's daughter's visit, survived the night early in the week when Janice told Anna she did not like what was going on between her mom and me. It seemed her mom always had to take care of someone.

"She doesn't know," I told Anna, "the closeness, all the little ways we have. It must be overwhelming to her. She has no model for our kind of relationship."

One morning toward the end of Janice's stay, I came out of my room and found Janice, Timothy, and Anna at the breakfast table, their talk heavy with sighs and long silences. Anna was crying, asking Janice again and again, "What do you want of me?" an expression she often used with me. Janice and Timothy were talking to Anna, comforting her as only they might, about her life, her running around, her not knowing what she was doing: selling the house or not, getting her Ph.D. or not, being always anxious and worried, never being there enough, never feeling she had her life in order. They were reassuring her yet being gently critical. She heard them and I think this affected how she was with me later.

After Janice left, Anna told me I had been "good" during her visit. I was careful to stay out of her way when she wanted time with her mother.

"Not good," I explained to Anna, noticing her surprise. "It didn't take any effort. I understood her. I understood her when she argued with you, when she said she'd been taking care of you since she was nine. She has the same sort of delicacy you have. Her emotions are so on the surface."

Two weeks after Janice left, Tim left too, after planting the yard with grass, refinishing the dining room table and chairs, and insulating the broad front windows that looked out on the mountain. When he left, Anna and I were again alone in the house, and I was determined to be calm, to be even, not to let things upset me as they had.

The morning after Tim drove off, my puppy, as if in desperation, dug huge holes in the lawn Tim had newly planted. Anna, looking out at the yard, spoke to me through her tears, "I'll never have a lawn."

Part Three

Difficulty Separating

VII: "I MISSED YOU"

That summer, amidst the comings and goings of Anna's children, there was a week when Anna left on a camping trip and I was alone in the house. At the start of that week, I was angry and by the end, I was simply afraid. The house, when she was gone, felt empty, as did a space near the core of my life.

The first day Anna was gone, I walked through the house crying, not knowing what to do with myself. I felt unsure of whether to close Anna's bedroom door—whether to close it and wipe her out, as Marc had once done in closing mine, or whether to keep it open, at least a crack, for some glimpse of a ghost of her being. I did not know how to go about being alone in that empty house. I turned on the television and lay there in front of it. I turned it off. I wrote Anna a note saying that I was angry she had fought with me the night before she left, itemizing my issues with her. I put it in her empty purse that sat on the counter in the kitchen, a kind of mailbox. Then I went into my room, sat in my chair, and felt a pain inside like some scourge, like an inner time bomb. I wanted to run, wanted someone to take care of me. Yet I was too tired to move. I picked up the phone and cried into it and hung it up.

That evening, a friend came to visit and I managed to hold back my tears as I made us dinner. When later we lay in bed together, I thought all the while of Anna. After my friend had left, I sat up by myself and was calmer. I thought of Anna on her camping trip with the group she had joined, riding down the river on a raft, thought of her in the night with the bugs and the dark, talking to people. I thought of her as she had been at home the night before: stern, cold, distant, not wanting to be a good mother to me. I had a headache and put my hand to it and finally turned out my light and went to sleep.

The next morning when I woke, I still had the headache and I did not want to get out of bed. So I stayed there for half the day, taking pills, drinking coffee, smoking cigarettes. I did not clean up the house, or feed the dogs or my cat or the horses next door. I did not want to take care of anything. I only wanted my head to stop hurting and not to cry. I wished that my crying would be over, that Anna would never come back, that I did not want a mother. I put on my dark glasses and lay in bed naked. Then, after a while, I took them off and was shocked by the brightness of the day outside. I lay waiting for it to go away, waiting for night.

After a few hours of waiting, a mother emerged from inside of me and started talking to me. She took me into the kitchen to get pills and juice. She took my cigarettes away and told me she would go with me to do things around the house—to take a shower and feed the horses and do the dishes and put my clothes away. She told me I could lie down again, but now my head was hurting too much and if I lay there, all I would feel was pain. She said to me that I was not alone; I would not have to do all these things by myself, she would be with me and watch my steps and sympathize with me for how hard it was. She would watch out for me, and if I felt too tired, she would sit down with me, or come back and lie with me on my bed.

I said to this mother no, I don't want to do anything. But finally I agreed to try, although I was still very tired, and my head hurt and walking around seemed like being in a dream. The house was so strange, so empty. I kept having visions of Anna on the raft and by the river.

I wanted to forget her, but, of course, I could not. I wanted to talk about Anna to the part of me that was the mother, to have her reassure me. But this mother of mine was the silent type. The only advice she had for me was that I should try not to be so angry. It was all right, she told me, to act in a dream while Anna was gone. The dream was a protection, a way to feel safe. And my anger was not at all safe.

I cried the second night after Anna was gone, and the third night before I went to sleep, though my crying was not as bad as at first. I woke each day later than usual, and went to sleep earlier. In the mornings, I was very slow and I did not want to move. The house was so empty, the phone barely rang, even the animals were more quiet than usual.

As the week went on, I began to feel better. I spent more of the time in my chair working. Sometimes the mother part of me took my cigarettes away, and sometimes I got up and fetched them back. I sat peacefully with my puppy and cat and Anna's dog sleeping in a circle at my feet.

In the middle of the week, I took a long walk, taking the dogs for a swim in the irrigation ditch, getting some sun. For I did not want Anna to come home and find me pale. I wanted her to find me healthy and strong. And this was different from how I had felt at first, when I wanted her to find me starving and sick, my face red and swollen from my tears. I wondered what would happen if I began to eat more, though this last thought scared me. For I did not want to be bigger.

I thought of Anna often. I thought about how the mosquitoes must be bad and how it would not be comfortable when there was a storm, how, much of the time, she would be wet. I decided finally I did not want to be on her trip, where, up until then, I had felt I did.

Yet I worried that I would look like less to her when she came back because I had not been with her, or climbed a mountain, or adventurously hiked into the woods while she was gone. I feared she would not love me.

The day before her return, I felt extremely helpless. I worried that we would get on as badly after she came home as we had the night before she left. I went to the grocery and bought a few things—watermelon, because Anna liked it, milk and bread, more scotch. I washed the dishes that had accumulated all week and vacuumed the house and thought back on the start of Anna's being gone. I wondered if I was better enough now. I was afraid I would not be able to manage my feelings when Anna returned. I would become too angry. I so wanted to see her, to consult her face for a reflection of what mattered between us.

That night, I looked in the mirror at my own face, which now showed signs of sun. At least I would not seem pale when I finally met Anna. I was healthier now, getting exercise each day, smoking fewer cigarettes. I was healthier but more afraid than I had been when Anna left. Late that night, I went to bed knowing the hours could now be counted. My legs felt very tired from my long walks with my puppy. I wrote a note to myself before I slept: "Dear little one, dear child: You are not as young as you seem in your thirty-four-year-old body, but younger than most your age, deceptively young. Little one, child, motherless so much of the time, you forget your own resolve to mother yourself."

The next morning, I woke wanting nothing but to see Anna. I drove into town to pick her up, but I could not find her group. No one was there in the parking lot, no travelers back with their bags. Late in the afternoon, I finally caught up with Anna back at the house. I found her showing the people who had given her a ride the outside of the house, for she had not taken a key. I let them in and sat at the dining room table smoking a cigarette, waiting. Anna looked marvelous. She was sunburnt, her face many different colors, there was dirt under her nails. She stood straighter than she had before she left. Her legs, in her sneakers, seemed planted more firmly on the ground. After the others had gone, she turned just inside the front door and hugged me, a long hug, and I felt not nearly as afraid as I had been.

We poured drinks and came into the living room, where I lay on the couch across from her. I heard about her days on the river, glad she was back, though all the time listening as if with a third ear for things she might say that would hurt me. I smiled as if relaxed but was wary, withdrawn, careful with my words, not sure if she was friend or enemy. When abruptly, breaking her own train of conversation, Anna looked at me and said she had missed me on her trip, missed me very much, wished that I had been there with her, I finally felt reassured. "I never thought I would say this," she added, looking a bit incredulous, "but I missed you as reality. You, my crazy friend, you are the most real."

Then I told her about my own week and it seemed not to surprise her—that I had been lost, sad, angry, wandering the house as a cave, that I had wished her to be sorry for having upset me the night before she went away, for leaving with things so unsettled between us.

We talked quickly now, interrupting each other, wanting to share. There was too much to tell. I followed her into the bathroom when she was ready to take a bath and saw how differently she held her body, showed herself. "We washed in the river nude together," she said. "I was raised to hide everything. But the women on this trip were younger, they seemed to feel, 'why should you have to hide your nipples or your pubic hair?'"

She sat in the tub and I on the floor of her bathroom, each with a glass of scotch, Anna lathering her hair with shampoo while it was still dry, so running water would not interrupt our words.

After her bath, she got dressed to go out to dinner with Marc. I left the house not much later to spend time with friends. When I got back, Anna was sound asleep in her bed, her clothes, but for her pants, still on, breathing deeply, the door to her room open. I stepped over to where she lay and kissed her, but she did not move, did not even pause between her breaths. I kissed her on the ear, but she did not respond. So I left her and went into my own room, leaving my door open so I could hear her breathing, strange now in the house that, for a week, had been silent. I listened to Anna's breathing as I might my own and imagined her not as far away as the next room.

Yet she was far away, I thought, full of a trip I had not taken, drunk, most likely, to sleep so soundly, because of Marc perhaps, because of what she had to face on coming back. "The trip was good but it did not take care of my depression," she had told me. "I'm as scared of my life as I ever was. No one there really took care of me. Though they probably thought they did. People kept telling me they were 'proud' of me, for climbing the cliff when I was so afraid, and getting back into the raft each time I fell out. They kept telling me they were so proud. A woman my age, they kept saying. But something about it wasn't right."

"It didn't feel real?"

"No, it didn't. None of the people on the trip were like you. You don't live on the surface."

That night, I lay and listened to Anna's breathing and felt very much better. Things seemed fine again, as fine as they might be. Anna was back. Yet I was still afraid—afraid we might fight, that I would be hurt. I was aware that even her presence could not calm what seemed to need to churn inside me. She was back. But this did not take my sadness away, or what, by now, seemed to be my eternal loneliness in that house.

VIII: "IT WON'T STOP THE FEELINGS"

I was lying in Anna's arms, telling her of my feeling sad and alone. "I want to tell you about the sharks," she said. Then she told me a story of all the cells in my body. "Each one is fighting for life," she began. "Every cell in your body wants to live. Each one's like a shark, a survivor."

That night when I went in to say goodnight to her, she murmured "Remember the sharks" as I turned to leave.

I would not myself have called them sharks. Yet I did know I needed some faith in those weeks as I neared the end.

"What's inside you?" Anna asked me one evening as we sat together on the couch.

"A space. A space full of light."

"And what else?"

"There's a picture hanging on a wall. It's a painting thick with blue and brown. It's very rich; it's life."

"Remember that picture when you begin to feel sad. It's in you. It's your richness."

Anna and I got along well right after she came back from her camping trip. We were careful with each other. Then for several nights, she had to stay at her brother's house in town while he was away. I visited her there each evening, bringing dinner, talking, then leaving to come home, and on each of those nights my leaving was hard, reminding me of another leaving—the day I would finally drive off, with my puppy and cat, with all my things.

People were leaving Anna. Marc had gone, and then Janice and Tim. I would go soon.

"I feel I've never had the dream," I told her one evening, "some ideal of perfection with you, the golden orb."

"But you've had it," she said. "If you'll just let yourself see it."

I thought often about my leaving during those last weeks. I was restless. I had trouble working. I did not want to take up my pen and know the feelings I was having. I thought of other years and other places, how I had started, how I had left. One night in anger, I smashed up a folding chair that was in my room, which we had brought from Anna's office to replace the one Marc took. "You made me do it," I told Anna, but I knew she had not.

"Don't leave in anger," she said to me, holding my hand. "It won't stop the feelings. You'll have them out there—on the other side. And I won't be there to see you through them."

I bought a new chair to replace the one I broke. I filled in the holes my puppy had dug in the yard and sprinkled in grass seed and watered it, hoping against the odds that the grass would grow.

I spent hours with Anna, talking about nothing, watching television, just being near, avoiding, to the greatest extent possible, the start of any friction between us. I did not tell Anna how many of my days were spent with a great impatience to leave, how present were my dreams of driving off. For I did not want to be gone yet, did not want her to feel me gone.

There were little things that reminded me that I was still here, but which I preferred not to notice because of the feelings they raised: the brown and black Indian pot that sat on my table that Anna had brought me from a trip north to tell me she cared. There was my puppy, the way he kept digging in the yard, anxious and searching, and my cat, who kept bringing me lizards.

Anna checked with me one weekend before making plans with Marc. She spent more time at home now than she had in months. We still drove into town and back together, and she kept her word and we did not, except on rare occasions, talk of Marc. She held me when I felt I was a scared child, and she said that although she got tired when with me, she would never leave me, never let me go.

During this time, we stayed up late on some nights drinking and talking as we used to. I brought Anna a scotch one night in bed and she said she felt cared for. She came in and checked on me one evening, when she had many phone calls to make, to see how I was feeling, if I was angry. She told me she felt sad that I would go. I was moved when she offered to help me stop smoking, when she looked at me and smiled and late at night laughed, when she asked me for money for lunch one morning before she left for work, and when she asked if I felt she needed a haircut. Anna left the door to her room open now at night when she went to bed, and when I made dinner, she commented that it was good.

All these things were important. The reality of our living together went on with a subtle intensity. Yet I so often tried to forget, living in fantasies of a future that was still a month off.

I drove around and did errands during those last weeks and looked at my arms, now brown from the sun, and I looked at the clouds in the broad sky, and I imagined myself out of time, in some strange place, and I imagined myself in my body alone.

One morning, I screamed and cried in the shower and later told Anna.

"Speak to the child," she said to me, "the one who gets so angry when she feels she'll be abandoned. Hold her. Be her mother. Take care of her as your own."

Yet I felt I did not have whatever was needed to reach out, to hold that child. I feared her problems, I did not want to take them on.

"But they're yours," Anna said. "You can't stop them by getting rid of me, by killing your mother."

"Yes," I said to her, not quite accepting.

Yes, I felt I also had to say to this very drifting life I was in, a life less full of the kind of work I knew, and usually took comfort in, than it was full of waiting, of sorting, of settling what had passed before moving on to what would come.

"I'm here now," I said to Anna and to anyone else when they spoke of the short time I had left, the fact that I was going. "I am here," I believe I was saying all during that time. "I'm getting together some strength in my soul—for the trip, the next life. I am here as a woman whose clothes are familiar, who now knows how to tune her car, who must come home at night to feed her puppy.

"I have not gone yet. I am full of what a person who is leaving must be full of, not driven for a while to 'make it.' I am here, as naked and bare as the desert, as full of small flowers and sparse growing things that are green. I am here with very little to show for myself but the fact of my existence, and this must for a time be enough."

Yet it was, by far, an easier statement for me to make than to believe. "I'm not working," I wished to cry out to Anna, to let her know of my sense of failure of worth.

"But you are. Work, like love, has many different forms. They do not all appear on paper."

"You don't seem to understand," she said to me another night, "how hard it will be on me when you leave." She was starting to cry standing before the counter in the kitchen, resisting the arm I held out to comfort her, preferring to grieve alone.

IX: LEAVING

How I missed her on that long drive. I left her in the morning, left her standing there beside the house looking after me as my car pulled away, her gray dog beside her—the old man, the "grandfather," she used to say, comparing him to my puppy. She had cried earlier that morning, and I had cried, holding her as we embraced, one of the many times we simply held close during those last few days.

I thought of her on my drive, thought back on the month before, the times I had been so angry. "I don't want to be sad," I had told Anna, striking out into the air with my fists. "I'm afraid to be sad."

"You won't cry forever."

"I don't want to cry at all."

Yet I did on the drive, in bursts, and when it began to get dark, in full anguished sobs. I would miss Anna. I already did. Like a hole in my heart.

The month before, I had been angry so often. One night as Anna and I were driving back from town together in her car, I had yelled at her that I wished I had already gone, that if I were still here, I would ask to be let off by the side of the road. That night we went to bed without speaking. The next morning, I sought to leave the house without making up. I yelled something at Anna before I left. She locked the door after me, wanting to hear no more of it. When I turned to come back in, I found the heavy wooden door locked. I pounded my hand against it, making my small finger black and blue, until Anna opened the door and I was let in.

"I'm sorry," I said. "You don't deserve my anger."

"I accept your apology," she told me. Though a few nights later as we sat talking she mentioned not liking my placating her so often, my apologies. "I don't know any other way," I said.

On the drive now, I looked at my hand as if it alone would remind me, as if it were alive with all I had left.

Those days, those weeks before I drove off, how vividly they seemed still with me: the night I raged at Anna like a madwoman, telling her all she wanted was a man, a penis. I was full of the hate, the anger for what I could not be. Earlier that evening, we had been sitting in the living room quietly, Anna reading, sewing two ruby-colored pillow covers she had just run off for me on the machine. Something she said sent me into my anger and I did not know enough to feel it false, a cover for the sadness I so feared. The next morning, Anna herself became angry, gripping me by the shoulders as we stood in the kitchen, knocking my head against a cabinet. It did not hurt, mostly felt good, like a relief, that she was angry at last.

"I drink because of you. I'm depressed. My life is terrible. It's never been as bad as this past year," she said.

Her words condemned me, yet I felt they freed me. They were, at the time, what I wanted to hear.

Later as we sat in the living room, Anna read and cried; she cried each time I came into the room or walked near. She was free to cry.

"I'm very afraid," she said finally. "I'm sick to my stomach, I'm so afraid."

We talked then and the angry words said so often between us the past few months faded, were taken back as untrue. "When I say I want to kill you, I'm telling you I am involved, I won't draw away,"

Anna said thoughtfully. "You make me so angry sometimes, I feel I want to kill you. But I don't draw back. I have always wanted to help you."

"I know. I appreciate it. I hear when you say you want to kill me how much you love me."

"Come," she said, holding out her arms, motioning for me to sit beside her on the couch and lie down with my head in her lap, like a child. "You're my little girl and I love you. Whatever you do, I love you."

That night, she held me close in bed and cried and spoke, at odd moments, of her anger: "It's primitive. Here I am holding you, thinking of how I will miss you, then all of a sudden I want to dig my nails into you. I'm angry with you for leaving."

The next day, we spent hours sitting together, holding one another, talking about other things but crying intermittently, no other subject quite covering what was happening between us.

The night before I left, we slept together for one last time in Anna's bed. I did not sleep well, but it did not matter.

"I thought about doing this two nights ago," she told me, "but then you got so angry, you talked so strangely, I simply wanted to leave the house."

I drove on my first day away for long hours into the night with my black puppy and calico cat perched up on suitcases in the back seat of my car, so they could see out, see what I could not.

My car broke down once not long after I left. It stopped and would not start. I called Anna in tears, crying like a child, a baby swept too soon out into the world. She answered and was not angry at this my first failure, my first block too large. That night when I spoke to her from a motel room very far away, my tears were too much, no words could speak my loss, my sense of fear, the hardness I felt in the face of the world.

"I cried on and off, I cry a lot," I told her. "I don't want to cry. My puppy's not used to any of this. He hasn't peed once. He's never lived outside the desert."

I was driving and leaving Anna farther and farther behind.

"You're still here," she told me that night, and the next, and the next. "I keep expecting you'll just come in from the other room. I keep talking to you, waiting to tell you things when I get home."

"I drive as if you're next to me in the car. I do that too," I said. "I want to come home."

But, of course, I could not.

"I feel like an invalid," I told her on one of my calls several days later, "as if I had an injury, a great sore, and I need to go slow to recover."

"I tell myself," I told her toward the end of my first week, "I tell myself when I can't find a house or something goes wrong, I say, 'You are of value. You have value, in yourself, for who you are, apart from this.' I tell myself and it helps. You taught me this, Anna. You taught me to cherish myself."

And then I could hear her smile, from far away, over the phone. And I pictured her in bed and pictured the house and the things I missed: that long dirt road to the bottom of the hill surrounded on all sides by the rising mesa, the scrub brush, the sand glaring with the summer sun. I pictured the view of the mountain; the house itself, low, adobe-brown, merging into the sandy hillside; my waiting for Anna to come home, looking out the front kitchen window for her; Anna watching after me the morning I left, standing high on the hill beside the house, not moving, her tears streaming down her cheeks. She was wiping them away with the back of her hand. I saw her coming home, pouring herself a drink, and the two of us busy in the kitchen—she with her papers and bills, me taking out food from the refrigerator.

"Anna, how do you feel about grilled cheese? Do you want tomato or not?"

"No tomato. Just plain. My mother always made cheese sandwiches with tomato. But I don't like tomato much. I like mine plain."

Now from afar, I pictured us at night, on those nights we talked so long on the couch. I missed some peaceful time I did not know if I ever had with Anna, some time of being truly happy. I missed waking up and coming out to the kitchen, anxious about what Anna's mood would be, wishing her to tell me that she loved me. I missed the very first time I was a child with her, the specialness of it, the going back, the time I got my puppy and dropped him hard and she held me.

I missed the evening we went to the wedding reception and I jumped all the curbs and we spent the night out alone. That was actually after Marc moved in.

I missed my very early time with Anna: "I have these feelings," she once said to me.

"It's not because you're a woman," she later said.

I hate thinking of those weeks just before I left—how angry I was, how Anna seemed on edge too, wanting to make sure she was not involved with me in some of the old ways she had decided were wrong, the sexual ways that both drew us together and kept us apart.

"Come let me hold you." "I think of your breasts often."

"The animals," I told Anna on the phone. "I took them from their home without their knowing they would never come back. My cat was sitting in the sun and I took her up so quickly and put her in the box. My puppy didn't know."

"It's happening too fast," I told her on my first night away. "I've left. It's happening too fast for me."

She told me that, for her part, she was in shock.

"It's like a dream for me," I said, "like I'm walking around in a dream."

"For me too."

We talked long on the phone several times and at first I felt better, just to hear her say, "I love you." I felt the words. Then toward the end of the week, I began to feel angry, that we could talk, yet I was still gone, becoming increasingly out of touch with the small daily things, what she did with her time, how she felt.

"I'm sick, Susan," she said to me. "I have an awful sore throat and I keep getting chills."

"It's a fever," I told her.

"I'm in bed."

Her voice was small and weak and I was afraid. She talked one day of selling the house, of another she had seen. Then her plans seemed to change. "It would be too much," she said, "too many changes in a short time. I'll feel just like you, overwhelmed. But you know I always do."

And I had images of her in the house in the mornings, by herself, in her state of fear when facing the day. When one morning and then another, I awoke and was shaking for hours with my own dread, I thought of Anna, wanted to call her, and did not. What could she do? I was far away, living in California, staying with a friend, unsettled as I ever had been, dressed but somehow raw, still the child half raised, half covered, not strong enough yet to face the world.

"Anna, I miss you. I want you here. I'm alone without you. So very alone. No one here really knows. They don't know I'm a child. They don't know how much you were my mother. They don't know how bad I was."

"Anna, I don't know if what we did was okay. All the fighting, how could it be good? I was such a bad little girl. And you were sometimes bad to me too. Anna, we were crazy part of the time, the best part. Anna, I'm very confused."

"Dear Susan," she wrote me during the first week I was gone, "I'm quite sick. I miss you."

"I gave my puppy and my cat away," I told her. "They're staying with someone while I look for a house."

"Anna, I don't have a home anymore. Anna, I don't—"

She called one night late and I wasn't home, to tell me she was feeling better, so I should not worry. Yet I worried nonetheless, that her life, whether she was sick or well, was increasingly beyond me, that she was a small voice in the middle of the country, that I had moved on, moved back, that I never again would be in touch with the child within myself in the way I most wanted, never love as I had.

"Anna?"

"Yes."

"Do you miss me?"

"I miss you very much."

For months, I lived moving from place to place, not unpacking, not happy in any new home. I continued to speak with Anna on the phone and occasionally when I hung up, I felt all right but mostly I did not. Anna's voice was small so far away, and I was small. I took care of my puppy. He would feel abandoned if I was away from him for long. He would greet me by jumping up high all over me in his old hysterical way whenever I drove up after having left him for a while.

It was hard to find a place to live. No one seemed to want me and my puppy, me and my child. I did not seem to want my child. I did not want to feel as I had with Anna, for fear the feelings would recall her, as they sometimes did late at night, when I was alone and I cried out in pain, wanting her, wanting a mother. In the days, I worked. In the nights, I thought about my child. I wished Anna would burn in some huge fire. I wished I would burn.

"Anna, why do you say that?" I asked her on the phone.

"Because you do. You badmouth me to people."

"I don't."

"Yes you do. You want them to believe that no one has been good to you, that you're all alone and abandoned so they will befriend you."

"I didn't know. Maybe I do. I'll watch myself."

Even then I was appeasing her, fearing to lose her, unsure of my view of what was real between us.

"I want to tell you about Anna," I wanted to say to someone. "I want to tell you—"

Conclusion

THIS BOOK BEGAN WITH A MEMORY of searching for a summer camp of my youth and has ended with a dramatic account of an intimate relationship that stays with me vividly still. In stories and small dramas, I have described changing geographic landscapes—a camp by a lake, a national seashore after a fire, a threatened pine tree in the yard behind mine, a trip down the California coast. I have evoked inner visions of fleeting lesbian landscapes—at a folk music festival, in a Mexican restaurant, in the classroom, and in bed. In several explorations of blindness and sight, I have described how my loss of eyesight has challenged me to see differently—initially when I first sensed I had a "fire" in my eyes, then as I learned to experience the world of a desert wildlife refuge in a new way, and finally as I recovered from a car accident and had to acknowledge, more than ever before, my increasing blindness. In my intimate portrait of my relationship with Anna, I have detailed a dramatic emotional liaison that marked my life and helped me to understand my needs.

In all of these stories, I have focused on telling the truth and prizing inner sight. I have painted my canvases with much detail, seeking to capture often invisible realities. When I began writing *Things No Longer There,* I knew only that I was distressed by changes in outer landscapes that had once been special to me. In the end, I found that my inner visions were more important than my external losses.

For me, this book has been an adventure in inner vision. When I think of the many stories here, I see an exhibit hall in a museum with pictures framed on the walls. These are pictures I can no longer see with my eyes, but when I look at them, dark and blurred in their frames, I see something vibrant and full of life, far more detailed than that portrait on the wall could ever be. The paintings in my mind are nuanced, full of gestures, in many colors and kinds of light, rich in emotional memories. There's a crane taking flight, a bright orange-pink sunrise, a small red car, the face of my lover youthful forever, my black dog with very soft fur. I see again the sweep of a beach at Half Moon Bay and the teeming marsh at Pescadero, feel the chill of green jello served by a white-frocked woman at a Mormon wedding. I feel the lure of a woman older than me who welcomed me into an adobe home in the desert back when I needed her. I see an expansive sky and a mountain through a window in a house on a mesa, and I see myself driving away, but looking back.

As I embark now on a new reality, walking off into a world of increasing blindness, I value all the more my internal imagery—the stories I tell myself, the inner humor, the detailed portraits I keep. I am finding my way without many of the visual clues I am used to, yet I am keeping my bearings, following my inner line of sight. I hope I will long remember lessons I have learned from this book about valuing inner visions, for these are the portraits that matter, these vibrant personal stories. I hope the reader, too, will value, all the more, the pictures on her inner walls.

Bibliographic Notes

Bibliographic Notes

I have long had a debt to authors whose works encourage the use of a personal female voice as a route to new kinds of knowledge. As I worked on *Things No Longer There: A Memoir of Losing Sight and Finding Vision,* the following works encouraged my use of my own voice in addressing broader themes: Marjorie L. DeVault, *Liberating Method: Feminism and Social Research* (Philadelphia: Temple University Press, 1999); Joan Didion, *The White Album* (New York: Simon and Schuster, 1979) and *Slouching towards Bethlehem* (New York: Washington Square Press, 1968); Estelle B. Freedman, *Maternal Justice: Miriam Van Waters and the Female Reform Tradition* (Chicago: University of Chicago Press, 1996); Barbara Laslett and Barrie Thorne, eds. *Feminist Sociology: Life Histories of a Movement* (New Brunswick, N.J.: Rutgers University Press, 1997); Nancy Mairs, *A Troubled Guest: Life and Death Stories* (Boston: Beacon, 2001), *Voice Lessons: On Becoming a (Woman) Writer* (Boston: Beacon, 1994), and *Plaintext: Deciphering a Woman's Life* (New York: Harper and Row, 1986); Laurel Richardson, *Fields of Play: Constructing an Academic Life* (New Brunswick, N.J.: Rutgers University Press, 1997); and Verta Taylor, *Rock-a-by Baby: Feminism, Self Help, and Postpartum Depression* (New York: Routledge, 1996). In sociology, I am indebted to the work of Norman Denzin, including *Performing Ethnography: Critical Pedagogy and the Politics of Culture*

(Thousand Oaks, Calif.: Sage, 2003) and *Interpretive Ethnography: Ethnographic Practices for the 21st Century* (Thousand Oaks, Calif.: Sage, 1997).

In the field of lesbian studies, I found the following works particularly relevant to my themes of lesbophobia and lesbian invisibility: Dorothy Allison, *Skin: Talking About Sex, Class and Literature* (Ithaca, N.Y.: Firebrand, 1994); Gloria Anzaldúa and Analouise Keating, eds., *This Bridge We Call Home: Radical Visions for Transformation* (New York: Routledge, 2002); Lucy Jane Bledsoe, ed., *Lesbian Travels: A Literary Companion* (San Francisco: Whereabouts Press, 1998); Meg Daly, ed., *Surface Tension: Love, Sex, and Politics between Lesbians and Straight Women* (New York: Simon and Schuster, 1996); Elana Dykewoman, *Moon Creek Road* (Denver: Spinsters Ink Books, 2003); Lindsey Elder, ed., *Early Embraces: True-Life Stories of Women Describing Their First Lesbian Experience* (Los Angeles: Alyson Publications, 1996); Lillian Faderman, *Naked in the Promised Land: A Memoir* (New York: Houghton Mifflin, 2003); Marilyn Frye, *Willful Virgin: Essays in Feminism* (Freedom, Calif.: The Crossing Press, 1992) and *The Politics of Reality: Essays in Feminist Theory* (Freedom, Calif.: The Crossing Press, 1983); Ellen Lewin, ed., *Inventing Lesbian Cultures in America* (Boston: Beacon, 1996); Marijane Meaker, *Highsmith: A Romance of the 1950s* (San Francisco: Cleis Press, 2003); Beth Mintz and Esther D. Rothblum, eds., *Lesbians in Academia: Degrees of Freedom* (New York: Routledge, 1997); Lisa C. Moore, ed., *Does Your Mama Know? An Anthology of Black Lesbian Coming Out Stories* (Decatur, Ga.: RedBone Press, 1997); Joan Nestle, *A Fragile Union: New and Selected Writings* (San Francisco: Cleis Press, 1998) and *A Restricted Country* (Ithaca, N.Y.: Firebrand, 1987); Esther Newton, *Margaret Mead Made Me Gay: Personal Essays, Public Ideas* (Durham, N.C.: Duke University Press, 2000); Carla Trujillo, ed., *Living Chicana Theory* (Berkeley, Calif.: Third Woman Press, 1998); Jacqueline S. Weinstock and Esther D. Rothblum, eds., *Lesbian Friendships: For Ourselves and Each Other* (New York: New York University Press, 1996); Vera Whisman, *Queer by Choice: Lesbians, Gay Men, and*

Bibliographic Notes

the Politics of Identity (New York: Routledge, 1996); and Bonnie Zimmerman and Toni A. H. McNaron, *The New Lesbian Studies: Into the Twenty-First Century* (New York: The Feminist Press at the City University of New York, 1996).

Within disability studies, I am indebted to the following writings for helpful guideposts: Sally Hobart Alexander, *Do You Remember the Color Blue? And Other Questions Kids Ask about Blindness* (New York: Viking, 2000) and *Taking Hold: My Journey into Blindness* (New York: Macmillan, 1994); Victoria A. Brownworth and Susan Raffo, eds., *Restricted Access: Lesbians on Disability* (Seattle, Wash.: Seal Press, 1999); Susan K. Cahn, "Come Out, Come Out Whatever You've Got! or, Still Crazy after All These Years," *Feminist Studies* 29: 1 (2003): 7–18; Eli Clare, *Exile and Pride: Disability, Queerness, and Liberation* (Cambridge, Mass.: South End Press, 1999); G. Thomas Couser, *Recovering Bodies: Illness, Disability, and Life Writing* (Madison: University of Wisconsin Press, 1997); Susan Crutchfield and Marcy Epstein, eds., *Points of Contact: Disability, Art, and Culture* (Ann Arbor: University of Michigan Press, 2000); Mary Felstiner, "Casing My Joints: A Private and Public Story of Arthritis," *Feminist Studies* 26:4 (2000): 273–285; Michelle Fine and Adrienne Asch, eds., *Women with Disabilities: Essays in Psychology, Culture, and Politics* (Philadelphia: Temple University Press, 1988); Beth Finke, *Long Time, No See* (Urbana: University of Illinois Press, 2003); Kenny Fries, *Body, Remember: A Memoir* (Madison: University of Wisconsin Press, 2003); Kim Q. Hall, ed., "Special Issue: Feminist Disability Studies," *NWSA Journal* 14:8 (2002); Georgina Kleege, *Sight Unseen* (New Haven: Yale University Press, 1999); Stephen Kuusisto, *Planet of the Blind: A Memoir* (New York: Dial, 1998); Nancy Mairs, *Waist-High in the World: A Life among the Nondisabled* (Boston: Beacon, 1996); Robert McRuer and Abby Wilkerson, eds., "Desiring Disability: Queer Theory Meets Disability Studies," *GLQ* 9:1–2 (2003); Rod Michalko, *The Two-in-One: Walking with Smokie, Walking with Blindness* (Philadelphia: Temple University Press, 1998); Frances Lief Neer, *Dancing in the Dark* (San Francisco: Wildstar Publishing,

1994); Shelley Tremain, ed., *Pushing the Limits: Disabled Dykes Produce Culture* (Toronto: Women's Press, 1996); and Susan Wendell, *The Rejected Body: Feminist Philosophical Reflections on Disability* (New York: Routledge, 1996).

Discussions of vision and of the functioning of the human eye that relate to my themes are: Gary H. Cassel, Michael D. Billig, and Harry G. Randall, *The Eye Book: A Complete Guide to Eye Disorders and Health* (Baltimore: Johns Hopkins University Press, 1999); Ian Heywood and Barry Sandywell, eds., *Interpreting Visual Culture: Explorations in the Hermeneutics of the Visual* (New York: Routledge, 1999); Donald D. Hoffman, *Visual Intelligence: How We Create What We See* (New York: Norton, 1998); and Stephen E. Palmer, *Vision Science: Photons to Phenomenology* (Cambridge, Mass.: MIT Press, 1999).

My previous studies developing a personal feminist sociology are: *The Family Silver: Essays on Relationships among Women* (Berkeley: University of California Press, 1996); *Social Science and the Self: Personal Essays on an Art Form* (New Brunswick, N.J.: Rutgers University Press, 1991); *The Mirror Dance: Identity in a Women's Community* (Philadelphia: Temple University Press, 1983); and *Hip Capitalism* (Beverly Hills, Calif.: Sage, 1979). A version of Chapter 5, "Half Moon Bay," appeared as "Things No Longer There: Half Moon Bay," in *Qualitative Inquiry* 7:6 (2001): 801–807.